EMQs for the MRCS Part A

EMQs for the MRCS Part A

Mr Sri G. Thrumurthy MBChB(Hons), MRCS
Core Trainee in General Surgery
London Deanery, UK

Miss Tania S. de Silva MBChB, MRCS(Ed)
Specialty Registrar in General Surgery
Sheffield Teaching Hospitals NHS Trust
Sheffield, UK

Mr Zia M. Moinuddin MBBS, MRCS
Specialty Registrar in General Surgery
Central Manchester University Hospitals NHS Foundation Trust
Manchester, UK

Professor Stuart Enoch MBBS, MRCS(Ed), PGCert (Med Sci), MRCS(Eng), PhD
Clinical Director, Centre for Study of Wound Care and Burns
Visiting Professor, Department of Biomedical Research Noorul Islam University, India
Director of Education and Research, Doctors Academy, Cardiff, UK

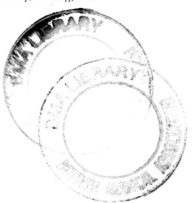

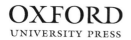

OXFORD
UNIVERSITY PRESS

OXFORD

UNIVERSITY PRESS

Great Clarendon Street, Oxford OX2 6DP
United Kingdom

Oxford University Press is a department of the University of Oxford.
It furthers the University's objective of excellence in research, scholarship,
and education by publishing worldwide. Oxford is a registered trade mark of
Oxford University Press in the UK and in certain other countries

British Library Cataloguing in Publication Data
Data available

ISBN 978-0-19-964564-0

DEDICATION

To my father and my greatest role model, Thrumurthy; to my loving mother,
Sobanah; to my wonderful wife, Ayishwarriyah; and to my baby sister, Sasha,
for their unconditional love and endless support. To Mr Muntzer Mughal,
for his relentless inspiration.

SGT

To my parents for their love and tireless support.
To Amit, for his endless patience and support over the years.
To Aiya, with love.

TSdS

To my parents, wife, and brothers for their constant encouragement and support.

ZMM

To Sri Thrumurthy, the lead author of this project, whose focus, passion and enthusiasm
helped us compile this resource; this endeavour would not have materialised
without his great commitment and motivation.

SE

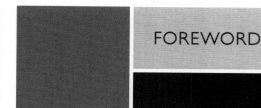

FOREWORD

As is well known, the I-MRCS Examination (the Intercollegiate Membership Examination of the Surgical Royal Colleges of Great Britain and in Ireland), comprises two parts:

Part A—Multiple Choice Questions (Written)

Part B—Objective Structured Clinical Examination (OSCE).

Part A is further subdivided into two papers: Paper 1, which is a test of knowledge in the Applied Basic Sciences, and Paper 2, which is an assessment of knowledge and competence in the Principles of Surgery-in-General.

As things stand, Paper 2 of the I-MRCS is made up exclusively of Extended Matching Questions (EMQs). This variety of multiple choice question is now recognized as an adequately validated, critically-evaluated, and well-established assessment tool, and regarded by educationalists as a reliable and discriminating method of assessing an examinee's command of applied knowledge. Conducted appropriately, the EMQ has the potential, also, to test higher order thinking. The EMQ format has for a number of years been embraced enthusiastically by the United States Licensing Examinations system and by the American Board examinations in various surgical and non-surgical specialties. The EMQ format is now being increasingly adopted and used in several postgraduate medical and surgical diploma examinations in the UK.

EMQs for the MRCS Part A by Thrumurthy, de Silva, Moinuddin, and Enoch is a very timely and worthy addition to every pre-MRCS surgical trainee's book shelf. Having taken on what can only be described as a herculean challenge, the authors have acquitted themselves with much credit. A great deal of thought, patience, diligence, and effort has gone into composing a most impressive collection of diverse EMQs. The EMQs have been classified into four chapters, with 20 to 25 EMQ units in each chapter. Throughout, the questions are worded unambiguously and in simple prose. Collectively the hundred or so well-constructed EMQs sample an impressive breadth of the I-MRCS syllabus. To complement the rich range of EMQs in each chapter, are the detailed answers to the EMQs which make up the latter half of each chapter. All the answers are comprehensive, well-researched, and reflective of contemporary practice. Very evidently, Mr Thrumurthy and colleagues have expended much time and effort to ensure the accuracy of the information they have provided in the book.

I have no doubt at all that the Foundation and Core trainees intending to sit the MRCS examination, and for whom this book is primarily intended, will find in this little gem of a book a most useful guide, resource, and friend!

I congratulate Mr Thrumurthy and colleagues warmly on their splendid effort and I commend this book with unreserved enthusiasm to all surgical trainees preparing for the MRCS examination.

Professor Vishy Mahadevan MBBS PhD FRCS
Barbers' Company Professor of Anatomy
The Royal College of Surgeons of England, London

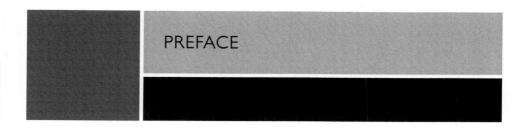

PREFACE

Major reform within the United Kingdom's postgraduate medical education system has necessitated a shift from the traditional true/false multiple questions of the old MRCS Part 1 examination to the 'single best answer' (SBA) and 'extended matching question' (EMQ) format used in the new intercollegiate MRCS Part A examination. Although a thorough understanding of the essential principles of surgery should be obtained from core textbooks and clinical experience, it is vital for candidates to actively recall, apply, and thereby reinforce their knowledge by attempting sample questions in the lead-up to the examination.

SBA MCQs for the MRCS Part A and *EMQs for the MRCS Part A* have been written to provide MRCS candidates with a series of questions preparing them for this new format. As the new format of the Part A paper de-emphasizes the traditional basic science disciplines and accentuates an integrated approach, these books will contain a substantial number of patient-based questions or clinical vignettes that will enable prospective candidates to test their ability to integrate key basic science concepts with relevant clinical problems.

Despite our attempt to comprehensively span the syllabus of the MRCS examination, it needs to be acknowledged that encompassing the full breadth and depth of all curricular topics is beyond the scope of this series. It is hence suggested that these books are used in conjunction with time-honoured surgical textbooks and used as a complementary resource rather than to supplement the reading material recommended by the Royal Colleges of Surgeons.

The detailed approach that these books undertake will not only serve MRCS candidates but will also be an appropriate revision aide for higher surgical trainees preparing for their intercollegiate speciality exit examinations. In addition, although the depth and breadth of this series' content surpasses that of typical undergraduate surgical curricula, these books will nevertheless be an ideal tool for the fervent medical student pursuing an 'honours' or 'distinction' grade in his or her surgical finals.

We sincerely wish all readers the very best of success in their surgical examinations and careers.

SGT
TDS
ZM
SE

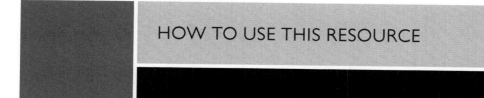

HOW TO USE THIS RESOURCE

Paper 1 of the new MRCS Part A examination comprises SBA questions relating to applied basic sciences whilst paper 2 consists of EMQs examining principles of surgery in general.

In keeping with the ethos of the examination, *SBA MCQs for the MRCS Part A* focuses intensively on the application of basic sciences (i.e. applied surgical anatomy, physiology, and pathology) to the management of surgical patients. *EMQs for the MRCS Part A* addresses topics relating to principles of surgery in general (i.e. perioperative care, postoperative management and critical care, surgical technique and technology, management and legal issues in surgery, clinical microbiology, emergency medicine and trauma management, and principles of surgical oncology). Each question has been mapped specifically to the MRCS syllabus as defined by the Intercollegiate Surgical Curriculum Project (ISCP). The explanation following each question aims to span the breadth and depth of the subject matter without overlapping with other explanations of similar themes. The diverse layout and level of detail included within the questions and their explanations will serve to help candidates tackle the MRCS Part A examination by allowing effective self-assessment of knowledge and quick identification of key areas requiring further attention.

We have formatted the questions to encompass various subtypes of questioning modalities to effectively guide candidates through the revision process. These modalities include 'clinical case' questions or 'clinical vignettes' (i.e. basic science applied clinically), positively-worded questions (i.e. requiring selection of the most appropriate of relatively correct answers), 'two-step' or 'double-jump' questions (i.e. requiring several cognitive steps to arrive at the correct answer), as well as factual recall questions (i.e. prompting basic recall of facts). The questions posed within these books will offer more thorough and detailed explanations than the majority of preparatory material currently available on the market. This is imperative because market research demonstrates that the vast majority of MRCS candidates are disappointed with the degree of description offered by most MRCS practice questions currently available (i.e. in books or within online question banks).

We are confident that this series, when used in conjunction with the recommended reading material of the Royal Colleges of Surgeons, will ensure the success of every candidate attempting the MRCS Part A examination.

SGT
TDS
ZM
SE

CONTENTS

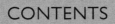

Abbreviations   xv

Chapter 1
Questions   1
Answers   20

Chapter 2
Questions   35
Answers   56

Chapter 3
Questions   71
Answers   92

Chapter 4
Questions   109
Answers   131

Index   151

ABBREVIATIONS

5-FU	5-fluorouracil
5-HIAA	5-hydroxyindoleacetic acid
AAA	abdominal aortic aneurysm
ABG	arterial blood gas
ABPI	ankle–brachial pressure index
ALP	alkaline phosphatase
ARDS	adult respiratory distress syndrome
ASA	American Society of Anesthesiologists
ASD	atrial septal defect
BiPAP	bilevel positive airway pressure
BMI	body mass index
BNP	brain natriuretic peptide
BP	blood pressure
bpm	beats per minute
CA	carbohydrate antigen
CAP	community-acquired pneumonia
CHART	continuous hyper-fractionated accelerated radiotherapy
Cl	chloride
CMV	controlled mandatory ventilation
COPD	chronic obstructive pulmonary disease
CPAP	continuous positive airway pressure
CPR	cardiopulmonary resuscitation
CRP	C-reactive protein
CT	computed tomography
CTPA	computed tomography pulmonary angiogram
CVP	central venous pressure
DCIS	ductal carcinoma in situ
DNA	deoxyribonucleic acid
DVT	deep vein thrombosis
ECG	electrocardiogram
ECMO	extracorporeal membrane oxygenation
ELISA	enzyme-linked immunosorbent assay

ERCP	endoscopic retrograde cholangiopancreatography
ER	(o)estrogen receptor
ESBL	extended-spectrum beta-lactamase
ESR	erythrocyte sedimentation rate
FAP	familial adenomatous polyposis
FAST	focused assessment with sonography for trauma
FBC	full blood count
GCS	Glasgow Coma Scale
GI	gastrointestinal
GKI	glucose, potassium and insulin (infusion)
GORD	gastro-oesophageal reflux disease
GP	general practitioner
GTN	glyceryl trinitrate
H	hydrogen
HAP	hospital-acquired pneumonia
Hb	haemoglobin
Hct	haematocrit
HER	human epidermal growth factor receptor
HLA	human leucocyte antigen
IL	interleukin
INR	international normalized ratio
IU	international units
JVP	jugular venous pressure
K	potassium
kPa	kilopascal
LFT	liver function test
MAWP	mean arterial wedge pressure
MCV	mean corpuscular volume
MRCP	magnetic resonance cholangiopancreatography
MRI	magnetic resonance imaging
MTC	medullary thyroid carcinoma
Na	sodium
NG	nasogastric
NICE	National Institute for Health and Clinical Excellence
NJ	nasojejunal
NSAID	non-steroidal anti-inflammatory drug
OGD	oesophagogastroduodenscopy
PaO_2	partial pressure of oxygen
PAWP	pulmonary artery wedge pressure
PCV	pressure-controlled ventilation

PE	pulmonary embolism
PEEP	positive end-expiratory pressure
PEG	percutaneous endoscopic gastrostomy
PET	positron emission tomography
PSA	prostate-specific antigen
PSV	pressure support ventilation
PVC	polyvinyl chloride
RBC	red blood cell
RCT	randomized controlled trial
RNA	ribonucleic acid
ROC	receiver operating characteristic
RTA	road traffic accident
SC	subcutaneous
SIRS	systemic inflammatory response syndrome
SpO_2	blood oxygen saturation
TNF	tumour necrosis factor
TMN	tumour, node, metastasis
TRALI	transfusion-related acute lung injury
USS	ultrasound scan
VAP	ventilator-associated pneumonia
VMA	vanillylmandelic acid
WCC	white cell count

1. Common surgical conditions and the subspecialties: Trauma and orthopaedics

A. Reiter's syndrome

B. Osteoarthritis

C. Intervertebral disc herniation

D. Metastatic disease

E. Rheumatoid arthritis

F. Paget's disease

G. Ankylosing spondylitis

H. Spinal stenosis

I. Multiple myeloma

J. Spondylolisthesis

For each of the following situations, select the single most likely diagnosis from the options listed. Each option may be used once, more than once, or not at all.

1. An 11-year-old girl is referred by her general practitioner (GP) to the Orthopaedic outpatient clinic with a 6-month history of lower back pain. Her parents state that she is a keen gymnast and believe that her symptoms may have been brought on by her undertaking excessive gymnastics activities. On examination, she is noted to have a mild degree of kyphosis and a palpable step deformity of her lumbar vertebrae. Straight leg raise is reduced and she experiences shooting pains along the distribution of the 5th lumbar nerve root when this manoeuvre is performed.

2. A 37-year-old forklift driver with no significant past medical history presents to the Emergency Department with severe lower back pain of sudden onset following lifting a heavy object whilst at work. He also complains of shooting pains down the back of his right buttock and thigh, but no bowel symptoms or urinary symptoms. Examination reveals paravertebral muscle spasm and a global reduction in spinal movements. Straight leg raise is restricted to 40° and also reproduces the shooting pains down his lower limb.

3. A 26-year-old man presents to his GP with a 6-week history of pain and stiffness in his lower back. He denies any previous trauma, although he believes that he may have sprained his back whilst playing squash a few weeks previously. Examination reveals a kyphotic posture, mild tenderness over the lower lumbar vertebrae, and restricted spinal movements in all directions. Plain radiography of the spine reveals an unstable fracture of the 4th lumbar vertebra. Initial serological investigations reveal a raised erythrocyte sedimentation rate (ESR) and positive human leucocyte antigen (HLA)-B27 antigen level.

4. A 22-year-old sailor presents to his GP with a 6-week history of a painful right knee and lesions on the soles of his feet. He also describes bilateral sore eyes and intermittent dysuria. Examination reveals a mild effusion within his right knee and generalized joint tenderness with restricted movements. Vesicles and pustules are noted over the soles of his feet, whilst examination of his eyes suggests conjunctivitis. Further questioning of the patient reveals that he had unprotected sexual intercourse eight weeks previously.

2. Common surgical conditions and the subspecialties: Skin, head, and neck

A. Acral lentiginous melanoma

B. Actinic keratosis

C. Amelanotic melanoma

D. Blue naevus

E. Keratoacanthoma

F. Lentigo maligna melanoma

G. Marjolin's ulcer

H. Nodular melanoma

I. Squamous cell carcinoma

J. Superficial spreading melanoma

For each of the following situations, select the single most likely diagnosis from the options listed. Each option may be used once, more than once, or not at all.

1. A 45-year-old policeman presents to his GP with a firm, symmetrically raised, and sharply delineated black patch over the volar aspect of his right distal forearm. Further questioning reveals that the lesion occasionally itches and bleeds.

2. An 85-year-old man presents to his GP with an irregularly shaped, brown patch over his left cheek. Examination reveals thickening and development of a discrete cutaneous nodule.

3. A 72-year-old farmer presents to his GP with a 2-month history of a rapidly-growing, solitary, fleshy, and elevated nodule over his left cheek. Examination reveals a firm, non-pigmented nodule with a hyperkeratotic core.

3. **The assessment and management of the surgical patient: Surgical history and examination**

   A. Anterior interosseous nerve
   B. Brachial plexus (lower cord)
   C. Brachial plexus (upper cord)
   D. Median nerve
   E. Posterior interosseous nerve
   F. Radial nerve (at the level of the axilla)
   G. Radial nerve (at the level of the mid-shaft of humerus)
   H. Radial nerve (at the level of the wrist)
   I. Ulnar nerve

   For each of the following situations, select the single most likely structure to be damaged from the options listed. Each option may be used once, more than once, or not at all.

   1. A 35-year-old athlete presents to his GP with a 12-hour history of wrist drop after falling off his cycle onto his left arm at high speed. He has no collateral injuries but cannot recall the exact details of the impact of his fall. Examination reveals altered sensation over the anatomical snuffbox, and an inability to extend the fingers at the metacarpophalangeal joints, of the left hand. All the reflexes in his left upper limb are normal.

   2. A 21-year-old medical student is seen in the Emergency Department after being hit by a cyclist on her left arm. She describes pain and severe weakness of her left hand. Examination reveals diminished power of extension at the left elbow, wrist and fingers, as well as sensory loss over the left dorsal forearm, and an absent triceps reflex.

   3. A 43-year-old prison warden is seen by the prison's doctor with a deep laceration to his right wrist from being slashed with a knife by an inmate. Examination reveals a weakness of finger abduction and pincer-grip, as well as diminished sensation over the ring and little fingers, on the affected side.

4. **Perioperative care: Postoperative complications**

A. Anastomotic leak
B. Chest infection
C. Deep venous thrombosis (DVT)
D. Intraperitoneal sepsis
E. Myocardial infarction
F. Pulmonary atelectasis
G. Pulmonary embolus (PE)
H. Systemic response to trauma
I. Urinary tract infection
J. Wound infection

For each of the following situations, select the single most likely postoperative complication from the options listed. Each option may be used once, more than once, or not at all.

1. A 35-year-old woman undergoes an uncomplicated laparoscopic cholecystectomy. When the patient is reviewed fourteen hours after the procedure, her temperature is observed to be 37.8°C and she describes mild pain and nausea. Her vital signs are otherwise normal and examination reveals a soft and mildly tender abdomen.

2. A 67-year-old man with no significant past medical history undergoes a right hemicolectomy for a Dukes' A colorectal tumour. He complains of significant pain forty-eight hours after the procedure, and is coughing up small amounts of white sputum. He is found to have a respiratory rate of 25/min, pulse rate of 105/min, temperature of 37.5°C and an oxygen saturation of 94% on room air. Examination of his chest reveals decreased expansion, dullness to percussion and reduced air entry to both lung bases.

3. An obese 55-year-old truck driver undergoes an elective total hip replacement. Ten days after his procedure, he is found to have a respiratory rate of 20/min, heart rate of 110/min, temperature was 37.8°C, and an oxygen saturation of 92% on room air. Examination of his chest, abdomen and operation site are largely unremarkable but his right calf is swollen and tender. A 12-lead electrocardiogram reveals atrial fibrillation and chest radiography is normal.

5. **Assessment and management of patients with trauma (including the multiply injured patient): Burns and skin loss**
    A. 27%
    B. 3510 mL
    C. 36%
    D. 4387 mL
    E. 45%
    F. 5850 mL
    G. Deep partial-thickness burn
    H. Full-thickness burn
    I. Superficial burn
    J. Superficial partial-thickness burn

For each of the following questions, select the single most likely answer related to the diagnosis or management of burns, from the options listed. Each option may be used once, more than once, or not at all.

1. A 42-year-old lady suffers burns to her skin from a house fire. The paramedics note that a large proportion of her burnt skin appears pale and leathery, and is numb to touch. What type of burn is this?

2. A 27-year-old fireman sustains multiple burns to his entire back, left arm and left thigh. The Emergency Department physician wishes to estimate the patient's total burn surface area prior to initiating fluid resuscitation.

3. A 62-year-old chef is assessed in the Emergency Department after sustaining multiple burns to his upper body during an accident in the kitchen. His total burn surface area is estimated at 36% (not involving the face, perineum, or thorax circumferentially) and his weight is 65 kg. The Emergency Department physician calculates the amount of fluid need for resuscitation in the first 12 hours using the Muir and Barclay formula.

6. **Basic and applied sciences: Microbiology**
    A. *Chlamydia trachomatis*
    B. *Clostridium botulinum*
    C. *Clostridium difficile*
    D. *Clostridium perfringens*
    E. *Clostridium tetani*
    F. *Escherichia coli*
    G. *Proteus mirabilis*
    H. *Pseudomonas aeruginosa*
    I. *Staphylococcus aureus*

For each of the following descriptions, select the single most likely causative organism from the options listed. Each option may be used once, more than once, or not at all.

1. These organisms are strictly aerobic, and generally opportunistic, causing infection in immunocompromised states (e.g. in patients with burns). They are commonly found in the environment.

2. These pathogens are often associated with the formation of struvite or staghorn calculi.

3. These anaerobic Gram-positive bacilli are the exotoxin-producing organisms that are commonly responsible for gas gangrene.

7. The assessment and management of the surgical patient: Clinical decision-making

A. Palliative therapy
B. Expectant management (following primary resection)
C. Curative chemoradiation
D. Adjuvant chemoradiation
E. Adjuvant chemotherapy
F. Curative chemotherapy
G. Anterior resection
H. Abdominoperineal resection

For each of the following situations, select the single most appropriate treatment from the options listed. Each option may be used once, more than once, or not at all.

1. A 45-year-old man undergoes a sigmoid colectomy for a tumour of the sigmoid colon. Histopathology reveals a well-differentiated adenocarcinoma of the colon infiltrating the submucosa, with no evidence of lymph node involvement. There is no evidence of distant metastasis.

2. A 60-year-old female undergoes a total colectomy and ileorectal anastomosis for a proliferative growth in the ascending colon, which was partially occluding the lumen. Multiple colonic polyps were incidentally identified during colonoscopy. Histopathological examination reveals a moderately differentiated adenocarcinoma of the colon infiltrating the pericolic fat. Seven out of nine lymph nodes demonstrate malignant spread and the entire colon has multiple adenomatous polyps. There is no evidence of distant metastasis.

3. An 88-year-old man presents to the surgical outpatient clinic with a 2-week history of abdominal distension and pain. Examination reveals jaundice and ascites. Computed tomography (CT) scanning reveals circumferential thickening of sigmoid colon with multiple liver metastases and pelvic deposits. The ascitic fluid cytology is suggestive of adenocarcinoma.

8. Perioperative care: Postoperative care

A. Caecostomy
B. Percutaneous endoscopic gastrostomy (PEG) feeding
C. Peripheral parenteral nutrition
D. Total parenteral nutrition
E. Special enteral feeding
F. Oral feeding
G. Nasogastric tube feeding
H. Jejunostomy feeding
I. Nasoenteric fine-bore feeding

For each of the following situations, select the single most appropriate feeding modality from the options listed. Each option may be used once, more than once, or not at all.

1. A previously healthy 22-year-old man is admitted to the neurosurgical ward after sustaining a moderate head injury from a high-speed road traffic accident. A CT scan of his head excludes any significant intracranial haemorrhage. Despite an initial Glasgow Coma Score of 12, he begins to exhibit progressive signs of recovery, and short-term nutritional support is being considered for him.

2. A 72-year-old man is admitted to the neuro-rehabilitation ward with dysphagia, dysarthria and left-sided hemiplegia after suffering a massive intracerebral bleed. He is deemed unfit for surgery due to a multitude of medical comorbidities, and will require long-term nutritional supplementation.

3. A 74-year-old woman is undergoing a Lewis–Tanner procedure for a stage III carcinoma of the distal oesophagus. She is not expected to undergo adjuvant chemoradiotherapy due to the curative nature of the surgical procedure. However, she has lost 15 kg in weight over the last four months (i.e. secondary to dysphagia and malignancy), and will require long-term nutritional support.

9. Professional behaviour and leadership: Medical statistics

A. Spearman's rank analysis
B. Student's t-test
C. Mann–Whitney U test
D. Kaplan–Meier analysis
E. Kolmogorov–Smirnov test
F. Wilcoxon signed-rank test
G. Fisher's exact test
H. Kruskal–Wallis test

For each of the following situations, select the single most appropriate statistical application from the options listed. Each option may be used once, more than once, or not at all.

1. A consultant surgeon wishes to use a non-parametric test to compare more than two groups of patients.

2. A professor of surgery is asked by her registrar to name a commonly used statistical test that provides correlation coefficients for non-parametric comparisons.

3. A medical student wishes to learn more about a commonly used statistical 'curve' that describes survival characteristics.

10. The assessment and management of the surgical patient: Differential diagnosis

A. Pelvic inflammatory disease
B. Crohn's disease
C. Acute appendicitis
D. Pelvic abscess
E. Acute cholangitis
F. Pyonephrosis
G. Pyosalpingitis
H. Subphrenic abscess
I. Acute cholecystitis

For each of the following situations, select the single most likely diagnosis from the options listed. Each option may be used once, more than once, or not at all.

1. A 23-year-old female presents to the Emergency Department with a 2-day history of severe lower abdominal pain and fever. She underwent a medical termination of pregnancy 10 days ago. Examination of the abdomen reveals severe suprapubic tenderness; and digital rectal examination reveals a soft, tender and fluctuant mass lateral to the rectum.

2. A 58-year-old diabetic female presents to the Emergency Department with a 24-hour history of severe right-sided loin pain and fever with chills and rigors. She is currently taking oral antibiotics for a recently diagnosed urinary tract infection. Examination reveals tenderness and a palpable mass within the right lumbar region.

3. A 45-year-old man presents to the Emergency Department with a 24-hour history of right upper quadrant abdominal pain, dyspnoea, pyrexia, and pain in his right shoulder tip. He recently underwent the repair of a perforated duodenal ulcer 3 weeks ago. Examination reveals a temperature of 38.3°C and severe tenderness over the right hypochondrium. Chest radiography reveals a right-sided pleural effusion.

11. Perioperative care: Postoperative complications

A. Hospital-acquired pneumonia
B. Pulmonary embolism
C. Pulmonary oedema
D. Acute respiratory distress syndrome
E. Community-acquired pneumonia
F. Type I respiratory failure
G. Type II respiratory failure
H. Exacerbation of chronic obstructive pulmonary disease
I. Acute severe asthma
J. Pneumothorax

For each of the following situations, select the single most likely postoperative complication from the options listed. Each option may be used once, more than once, or not at all.

1. A 70-year-old-man with a history of ischaemic heart disease and hypertension undergoes an open repair of his abdominal aortic aneurysm. On postoperative day 3, he develops pleuritic chest pain, a cough, and dyspnoea. Examination reveals tachypnoea, tachycardia, mild pyrexia, and reduced air entry in the right lung base. Arterial blood gas analysis reveals a pH of 7.35, pO_2 of 9.8 kPa, and pCO_2 of 5 kPa.

2. A 62-year-old-woman with a history of rheumatoid arthritis and ischaemic heart disease undergoes a right hemicolectomy for cancer of the ascending colon. On postoperative day 6, she develops sudden-onset dyspnoea, pleuritic chest pain, and a cough. On examination she is tachypnoeic, tachycardic, with slightly reduced air entry in the right base. Arterial blood gas analysis demonstrates a pH of 7.47, pO_2 of 8.5 kPa, and a pCO_2 of 3.5 kPa.

3. A 75-year-old-man with a history of ischaemic heart disease undergoes an emergency laparotomy and oversewing of a perforated duodenal ulcer. On postoperative day 2, he develops sudden-onset dyspnoea and tachypnoea. He remains apyrexial, and examination of his chest reveals bibasal crepitations on auscultation. Arterial blood gas analysis demonstrates a pH of 7.35, pO_2 of 8.2 kPa, and pCO_2 of 5.0 kPa.

12. Professional behaviour and leadership: Medical consent

A. Surgery cannot proceed
B. Surgery can proceed without consent from patient
C. Surgery cannot proceed without consent from patient
D. Second opinion and referral to the courts
E. Surgery can proceed with consent from parents
F. Surgery can proceed under the Mental Capacity Act
G. Consent from child is sufficient to deliver treatment
H. Consent is implied
I. Consent may be obtained from patient's partner

For each of the following situations, select the single most appropriate outcome from the options listed. Each option may be used once, more than once, or not at all.

1. A 45-year-old man is undergoing compulsory treatment on a psychiatric ward for a severe psychiatric illness. He develops acute abdominal pain and is diagnosed with a perforated duodenal ulcer. The surgeon and the psychiatrist agree that a laparotomy is the best treatment option. What is the consent process that should be followed?

2. A 23-year-old woman who is 28 weeks pregnant develops abdominal pain and is diagnosed with appendicitis. It is explained to her that appendicectomy is the best treatment given that the risks of fetal mortality and maternal morbidity are significantly higher with non-operative management compared to operative treatment. The patient understands this but still declines surgery. Her husband wants the operation to proceed but the patient still refuses surgery. What is the consent process that should be followed?

3. A 30-year-old man is brought to the Emergency Department, unstable and unconscious following a RTA. He is diagnosed with an expanding extradural haematoma and needs an urgent burr hole and craniectomy to evacuate the haematoma. His wife, who is by his side, refuses to agree to the operation. What is the consent process that should be followed?

4. A 12-year-old-boy presents to the Emergency Department with severe abdominal pain and generalized peritonitis. The surgeon explains to the parents that the boy requires an urgent laparotomy. The parents understand the risks and benefits of this but refuse to allow the boy to undergo major surgery for religious reasons. What is the consent process that should be followed?

13. The assessment and management of the surgical patient: Clinical decision-making

A. Arthrodesis
B. Cannulated screw
C. Dynamic hip screw
D. Full leg plaster cylinder
E. Hemiarthroplasty
F. K-wire fixation
G. Skeletal traction
H. Tension band wiring
I. Total hip replacement

For each of the following situations, select the single most appropriate procedure from the options listed. Each option may be used once, more than once, or not at all.

1. A 78-year-old osteoporotic female is brought into the Emergency Department having slipped and fallen on ice. Radiography of her hip reveals an undisplaced intertrochanteric fracture of her right femoral neck.

2. A 70-year-old woman with poor mobility and known postural hypotension sustains a fall while trying to get out of bed. She is brought into hospital with a shortened, externally rotated left leg. Radiography of the hip reveals an intracapsular fracture of the femoral neck with disruption of trabeculae and complete displacement of the femoral head.

3. A 50-year-old man is involved in a RTA. He is brought into hospital unable to weight bear. He is found to be haemodynamically stable with no open wounds or other injuries. The radiographs reveal a bicortical intracapsular fracture of the femoral neck with no evident displacement.

14. Perioperative care: Intraoperative care

A. Caecostomy
B. Hartmann's procedure
C. Jejunostomy
D. Loop colostomy
E. Loop ileostomy
F. Mucus fistula
G. Paul–Mikulicz procedure
H. Percutaneous endoscopic gastrostomy
I. Permanent end colostomy
J. Spout ileostomy
K. Stamm gastrostomy

For each of the following situations, select the single most appropriate procedure from the options listed. Each option may be used once, more than once, or not at all.

1. A 38-year-old solicitor has longstanding ulcerative colitis that has recently become refractory to medical treatment. She is keen to undergo surgery but is apprehensive about the need for a stoma. After preoperative workup, the surgeon recommends a restorative proctocolectomy and ileoanal pouch formation but advises the patient that she will need a temporary stoma for 8–10 weeks postoperatively.

2. A 72-year-old gentleman presents to the Emergency Department with a 12-hour history of painful abdominal distension and absolute constipation. Examination reveals no signs of peritonitis, and the patient is haemodynamically stable. Plain abdominal radiography reveals grossly dilated loops of large bowel, and an unprepared gastrografin enema reveals an obstructing lesion in the mid-sigmoid colon. A laparotomy is performed and a stoma is formed.

3. A 65-year-old gentleman with a history of poorly-controlled ulcerative colitis presents to the Emergency Department with a 6-hour history of acute-onset, severe abdominal pain. Examination reveals signs of generalized peritonitis. A laparotomy is performed following resuscitation, revealing faecal peritonitis secondary to a perforated sigmoid tumour. A sigmoid colectomy was performed, with the proximal segment exteriorized as an end colostomy. The surgeon then proceeds to work on the distal segment.

15. The assessment and management of the surgical patient: Appropriate prescribing

A. Aminoglycoside

B. Beta-lactam

C. Carbapenem

D. Cephalosporin

E. Fluoroquinolone

F. Macrolide

G. Sulphonamide

H. Tetracycline

I. None of the above

For each of the following situations, select the single most appropriate antibiotic therapy from the options listed. Each option may be used once, more than once, or not at all.

1. Used to treat Gram-negative sepsis, these antibiotics need to be administered intravenously or intramuscularly as they are not absorbed from the small intestine. They have a prolonged dosage interval and are known to be ototoxic and nephrotoxic.

2. These antibiotics are commonly prescribed for surgical prophylaxis, and are responsible for adverse side effects such as diarrhoea, nausea, rash, and pseudomembranous colitis.

3. These chemotherapeutic antibiotics are contraindicated in children, pregnancy, and in patients with epilepsy. They do not demonstrate a significant first-pass metabolic effect and bioavailability remains similar between oral and intravenous administration. They interact with the metabolism of warfarin, phenytoin, levothyroxine, and non-steroidal anti-inflammatory drugs (NSAIDs).

16. Perioperative care: Coagulation, deep vein thrombosis, and embolism

A. Early postoperative mobilization

B. Inferior vena cava filter

C. Lower limb venous duplex ultrasound scan (USS)

D. Omit all anticoagulation

E. Standard-dose prophylactic low-molecular-weight heparin

F. High-dose prophylactic low-molecular-weight heparin

G. Start warfarin until 5 days prior to operation then convert to heparin infusion until 6 hours prior to operation.

H. Treatment-dose low-molecular-weight heparin

I. Treatment-dose warfarin

For each of the following situations, select the single most appropriate management strategy from the options listed. Each option may be used once, more than once, or not at all.

1. A 45-year-old female with factor V Leiden deficiency is admitted for an elective day-case laparoscopic cholecystectomy.

2. A 55-year-old male is admitted for an elective cardio-oesophagectomy following neoadjuvant chemotherapy for gastro-oesophageal malignancy. He has recently been diagnosed with a small below-knee deep vein thrombosis (DVT) and has had two minor episodes of haematemesis.

3. A 65-year-old male with an early colonic tumour is electively admitted for a sigmoid colectomy. Whilst in hospital he becomes acutely short of breath. He undergoes a computed tomography pulmonary angiogram (CTPA), which confirms the presence of multiple small pulmonary emboli. The patient is subsequently commenced on heparin in anticipation for his surgery.

17. The assessment and management of the surgical patient: Differential diagnosis

A. Allergic conjunctivitis
B. Episcleritis
C. Scleritis
D. Keratitis
E. Corneal abrasion
F. Acute closed-angle glaucoma
G. Anterior uveitis
H. Subconjunctival haemorrhage
I. Infective conjunctivitis

For each of the following situations, select the single most likely diagnosis from the options listed. Each option may be used once, more than once, or not at all.

1. A 60-year-old diabetic man presents to the Emergency Department with a 2-hour history of sudden-onset, severe pain in his right eye. He also complains of some haziness in vision and vomiting. On examination, the right eye appears diffusely injected and hypersensitive to light. The pupil is mid-dilated and oval-shaped, and the cornea appears hazy. What is the likely diagnosis?

2. A 50-year-old woman with rheumatoid arthritis is seen in the Emergency Department with gradual-onset, bilateral severe eye pain, increased lacrimation and photophobia. Examination reveals diffuse redness in both eyes, with injection of the vessels in the deeper layer. The patient's and visual acuity are normal. What is the likely diagnosis?

3. A 40-year-old diabetic man presents with a painful and red right eye. Examination of the affected eye reveals circumlimbal injection, watery discharge and photophobia. The right pupil appears constricted and irregularly shaped, with blurred vision and decreased visual acuity elicited in the right eye. What is the likely diagnosis?

18. Perioperative care: Postoperative complications

A. 1–2%
B. 5–10%
C. 10–15%
D. 15–20%
E. 20–30%
F. 40%
G. 80%
H. 100%

For each of the following situations, select the single most likely risk of wound infection from the options listed. Each option may be used once, more than once, or not at all.

1. A 55-year-old female undergoes an emergency laparoscopic cholecystectomy for acute severe cholecystitis.

2. A 54-year-old diabetic male is admitted electively for an inguinal hernia repair with mesh fixation.

3. A 70-year-old male who undergoes an emergency laparotomy for peritonitis is found to have a perforated sigmoid diverticulum during surgery.

19. The assessment and management of the surgical patient: Differential diagnosis

A. Acute heparin-induced thrombocytopenic purpura

B. Acute hepatic failure

C. Acute respiratory distress syndrome

D. Disseminated intravascular coagulation

E. Fat embolism syndrome

F. Hepatorenal syndrome

G. Multiorgan dysfunction syndrome

H. Multiorgan failure

I. Systemic inflammatory response syndrome

For each of the following situations, select the single most likely diagnosis from the options listed. Each option may be used once, more than once, or not at all.

1. A 48-year-old farmer is brought into the Emergency Department having been run over by a tractor. On arrival he is found to be tachypnoeic, tachycardic, and confused. Examination reveals a widespread petechial rash and a fracture-dislocation of the mid-shaft of his femur. There are no neurological abnormalities. Chest radiography excludes haemothorax and pneumothorax but reveals bilateral pulmonary infiltrates.

2. A 75-year-old lady is admitted with a single episode of bloody diarrhoea and abdominal pain. She is investigated with rigid sigmoidoscopy when her symptoms subside, and is found to have chronically ischaemic bowel. Over the course of her admission, she becomes tachycardic, hypotensive and acidotic. Her urine output falls to 10 mL per hour and her serum urea and creatinine levels are found to be 35 mmol/L and 690 μmol/L respectively. She receives delayed fluid resuscitation but unfortunately, her oliguria and hypotension do not respond well to this.

3. A 63-year-old female is trapped in a house fire, suffering second-degree burns to 30% of her total body surface area. She is tachypnoeic and hypoxic on arrival to hospital, and is found to have soot and singed hairs within her nostrils. She responds poorly to supplementary oxygen in the Emergency Department. Chest radiography demonstrates bilateral pulmonary infiltrates.

20. Basic and applied sciences: Microbiology

A. *Staphylococcus aureus*
B. *Enterococcus* species
C. *Escherichia coli*
D. Coagulase-negative staphylococci
E. *Pseudomonas aeruginosa*
F. *Klebsiella pneumoniae*
G. *Enterobacter* species
H. *Proteus mirabilis*
I. *Candida* species
J. *Clostridium difficile*

For each of the following situations, select the single most likely causative organism from the options listed. Each option may be used once, more than once, or not at all.

1. This Gram-positive organism is part of normal skin and mucous membrane flora. 30% of adults carry this pathogen in their anterior nares. The organism is both aerobic and anaerobic in blood agar cultures.

2. This anaerobic organism is a common commensal of the gastrointestinal tract. It is a significant cause of nosocomial infections. This organism is intrinsically resistant to beta-lactams and aminoglycosides.

3. Certain antibiotics including lincomycin allow the colonization of this pathogen. Broad-spectrum antibiotics are the main cause. The bacteria produce exotoxins that cause gastrointestinal mucosal inflammation.

21. **The assessment and management of the surgical patient: Clinical decision-making**

A. Radiotherapy alone
B. Radiotherapy and chemotherapy
C. Letrozole (lifelong)
D. Radiotherapy and tamoxifen
E. Radiotherapy, chemotherapy, and tamoxifen
F. Chemotherapy alone
G. Letrozole for 5 years
H. Tamoxifen for 5 years
I. Neoadjuvant chemotherapy
J. Neoadjuvant hormone therapy
K. No further treatment required

For each of the following situations, select the single most appropriate therapy from the options listed. Each option may be used once, more than once, or not at all.

1. A 30-year-old lady undergoes a mastectomy and axillary clearance for a large, poorly-differentiated invasive ductal carcinoma. The tumour is found to be strongly ER ((o) estrogen receptor) positive but HER2 negative. What form of adjuvant therapy would be indicated in this patient?

2. An 84-year-old lady, who is a nursing-home resident with vascular dementia, presents to the breast clinic with a lump in her left breast. Examination reveals an irregular, hard lump in her left breast with evident skin tethering. A core biopsy of the lesion confirms an invasive ductal cancer. What further treatment would be appropriate for this patient?

3. A 34-year-old lady undergoes a wide local excision of a lump in her right breast. Histology confirms a high-grade ductal carcinoma *in situ* (DCIS) which is strongly ER positive. What further treatment would be indicated for this patient?

4. A 36-year-old lady undergoes a wide local excision of a 2 cm lump in her left breast. Histology confirms a low-grade DCIS and the tumour is strongly ER positive. What further treatment would be indicated for this patient?

22. Basic surgical skills: Closures

A. Catgut
B. Dexon®
C. Linen
D. Nylon
E. PDS®
F. Prolene®
G. Silk
H. Steel
I. Vicryl®

For each of the following situations, select the single most appropriate suture material from the options listed. Each option may be used once, more than once, or not at all.

1. A consultant surgeon describes to his medical student the advantages of a synthetic, braided, absorbable suture which elicits minimal tissue reaction and is hydrolysed within 56–70 days.

2. A vascular surgeon wishes to use a synthetic, monofilament, non-absorbable suture to perform an arterial anastomosis.

3. A consultant surgeon asks his scrub nurse for a suture to secure his abdominal drain in place. He tells his medical student that this is a natural, braided, non-absorbable suture that is rarely used for other purposes due to its nature of evoking a marked tissue reaction.

23. The assessment and management of the surgical patient: Clinical decision-making

A. Brain tumour
B. Breast cancer
C. Cervical cancer
D. Colon cancer
E. Head and neck cancer
F. Malignant melanoma
G. Prostate cancer
H. Sarcoma
I. Thyroid cancer

For each of the following modalities of radiotherapy, select the single most appropriate pathology to be treated by this form of radiotherapy from the options listed. Each option may be used once, more than once, or not at all.

1. Improved survival rates have been found with the use of continuous hyper-fractionated accelerated radiotherapy (CHART), which is given three times a day over 12 days.

2. Radioactive material such as caesium can be enclosed in impenetrable cases such as those made with platinum and inserted directly into the tissue to be irradiated, minimizing the effect of radiation on surrounding tissue.

3. Radioactive iodine-131 can be administered orally to be absorbed from the bloodstream by residual cancer cells that require ablation following surgical resection.

24. Basic surgical skills: Principles of sterilization

A. Irradiation
B. Hot ovens
C. Ethylene oxide
D. Autoclaves
E. Iodine
F. Gas plasma
G. Low-temperature steam
H. Sporicidal chemicals
I. Chemical disinfectants
J. Boiling water

For each of the following descriptions, select the single most likely form of sterilization from the options listed. Each option may be used once, more than once, or not at all.

1. This expensive method of sterilization is highly successful against bacteria, spores, and viruses. A toxic residue is left on the equipment, which therefore has to be stored for a period of time before it can be used.

2. This highly effective and economical procedure utilizes pressurized steam at a high temperature. For the procedure to be effective, the steam has to be in direct contact with the material requiring sterilization. This procedure is therefore unsuitable for heat-sensitive objects.

3. This method of sterilization is successful if used for a prolonged period. It is economical and suitable for heat-sensitive items. The most commonly used sterilizing agent for this method is 2% glutaraldehyde.

1. Answers: 1-J; 2-C; 3-G; 4-A

1. The signs and symptoms of this child are suggestive of lumbar spondylolisthesis. Spondylolisthesis refers to the anteroposterior displacement of one vertebra in relation to the vertebra below it. Isthmic spondylolisthesis is one type (of five) and appears to be a form of repetitive stress fracture; the incidence of this pathology is notably higher in teenage gymnasts and other athletes. It commonly occurs between the ages of 7–10 years. The signs and symptoms of spondylolisthesis include low back pain, hamstring spasm, 5th lumbar nerve root pain, and disturbance in the sagittal profile of the spine with an acute kyphosis. Neurological symptoms involving the lower limb may be observed in some patients. Examination may reveal a 'step' deformity along the line of the spinous processes. The ability to perform the 'straight leg raise' test may be reduced due to hamstring spasm, and radicular (i.e. involving the nerve root) neurological symptoms may be reproduced by this test. Lumbar spondylolisthesis may be managed conservatively with bed rest during acute attacks; and supporting corsets between attacks. In young adults or patients with disabling symptoms or evidence of marked neurological compression, operative treatment (i.e. spinal fusion to fix the unstable segment) is indicated.

2. This patient demonstrates the features of lumbar disc herniation (prolapse). This condition commonly occurs in fit, young adults usually when lifting heavy weight or whilst straining. A sudden, acute pain may be felt in the lower back, and this may be accompanied by shooting pains radiating to the buttock or down the leg along the distribution of the affected nerve root. Examination reveals paravertebral muscle spasm, often leading to a 'spinal tilt' and a global reduction in spinal movements. Straight leg raise is often restricted to <50° and performing this manoeuvre may reproduce the radicular symptoms. The management of this condition is largely symptomatic, with a proportion of patients requiring disc decompression for intractable symptoms or cauda equina syndrome.

3. This patient demonstrates the signs and symptoms of ankylosing spondylitis. Ankylosing spondylitis is predominantly observed in young adults and has a male preponderance (6:1). Patients typically present with symptoms of morning stiffness, backache, progressive loss of spinal movements (leading to kyphosis), and hyperextension of the neck (i.e. leading to the classical 'question mark' posture). Patients may occasionally present with unstable fractures following minor trauma. Plain radiography may reveal bony ankylosis of the intervertebral joints; ossification of the discs and the bony bridges between vertebrae (i.e. syndesmophytes) creates the classical 'bamboo spine' appearance with squaring of the vertebral bodies. Blood tests may reveal raised ESR, normochromic anaemia and positive HLA-B27 antigen. The treatment of ankylosing spondylitis is largely symptomatic, with simple analgesia and other immunomodulatory agents (e.g. sulphasalazine and TNF-alpha antagonists). Vertebral osteotomy may be used to treat severe flexion deformity, and total hip replacement to treat affected hip joints. It is essential for patients to maintain their mobility; postural training may help to previous serious deformities.

4. This patient's history and examination findings suggest the diagnosis of Reiter's syndrome. Reiter's syndrome (also known as sexually-acquired reactive arthritis) is a triad of urethritis, conjunctivitis (or iritis) and seronegative arthritis. The patient is typically of young age, suffering from a mono- or polyarthritis affecting the knees, ankles, feet and hands. Other musculoskeletal manifestations of Reiter's syndrome include sacroiliitis, which is commonly asymptomatic, plantar fasciitis, Achilles tendonitis, and calcaneal spur enthesopathy causing heel pain. Various other features of this condition include keratoderma blenorrhagica (brown, aseptic abscesses on the soles and palms), circinate balanitis (painless serpiginous penile rash), venereal non-gonococcal urethritis, conjunctivitis (usually bilateral and sterile), fever, malaise, cachexia and rarely, pleurisy or pericarditis. The management of the arthritis of Reiter's syndrome involves rest, immobilisation of the affected joints, aspiration of joint effusions, non-steroidal anti-inflammatory drugs and steroids. Physiotherapy is also of benefit to such patients. The urethritis and conjunctivitis are managed with antibiotics if evidence of infection is present; the keratodermia blenorrhagica may be treated with 1% hydrocortisone.

2. Answers: 1-H; 2-F; 3-E

Melanomas are malignant tumours of melanin-producing cells called melanocytes. 95% of melanomas are confined to the skin, while the rest occur primarily in extracutaneous sites (e.g. the eye, gastrointestinal or genitourinary systems, central nervous system, and lymph nodes). Metastasis occurs via superficial lymphatics to give satellite lesions; to regional lymph nodes via deep lymphatics; and via haematogenous spread to the lung, liver, and brain. Haematogenous spread usually follows lymphatic spread.

Malignant melanomas undergo two growth phases: radial and vertical, with vertical invasion being associated with a poorer prognosis. In order of prevalence, the five main subtypes of melanoma are: superficial spreading (70%), nodular (15%), lentigo maligna (5–15%), acral lentiginous (including periungual, 5%) and amelanotic melanoma (1%).

To date, the best prognostic indicator in stage I (i.e. non-metastatic) malignant melanoma is the Breslow thickness, which is measured in millimetres from the overlying granular layer of the epidermis to the deepest easily identifiable tumour cells with an ocular micrometer. As per Breslow thickness, the 5-year survival rates are:

- <1.5 mm (good—95%)
- 1.5–3.5 mm (intermediate—65%)
- >3.5 mm (poor—35%).

A less commonly used prognostic indicator is Clark's index, which corresponds to the histological level of invasion:

I: *in situ*; confined to epidermis
II: invasion of papillary dermis
III: filling of papillary dermis but no extension into reticular dermis
IV: invasion of reticular dermis
V: invasion of subcutaneous tissue.

Table 1.1 The 2010 Revised UK guidelines for the management of cutaneous melanoma

Breslow thickness	Excision margins
In situ	5 mm (to achieve complete histological excision)
<1 mm	1 cm
1–2 mm	1–2 cm
2–4 mm	2–3 cm
>4 mm	3 cm

The management of malignant melanoma involves an initial excision biopsy and histological examination. Surgery is commonly performed after biopsy, with the traditional width of excision being 3–5 cm. The revised UK guidelines for the management of cutaneous melanoma (2010) recommend the surgical excision margins listed in Table 1.1.

Superficial spreading melanomas and nodular melanomas are radioresistant but good results have been reported from radiotherapy for lentigo maligna melanoma. Involved regional lymph nodes are removed by block dissection; prophylactic lymph node dissection is rarely performed in the UK. Recurrent or deeply invasive tumours may respond to limb perfusion (i.e. arterially perfusing the affected limb with a cytotoxic agent, e.g. melphalan)—this reduces recurrence but may result in anaemia if the bone marrow is penetrated. Immunotherapy and hormonal therapy are currently being evaluated. Most patients are followed up for 10 years (i.e. 3-monthly for the first 2 years and 6-monthly thereafter).

1. Nodular melanoma is the most rapidly growing and aggressive subtype of malignant melanoma. It lacks the typical radial growth phase, and is usually seen on the trunk and limbs of patients aged 40–60 years (males > females). It has relatively little melanin and a rich blood supply. Patients usually present with a symmetrical, raised, firm, uniformly coloured, and frequently non-pigmented nodule which continue to enlarge and become more raised. Ulceration is common and indicates a poorer prognosis.

2. Lentigo maligna melanoma (Hutchinson's melanotic freckle) classically occurs in the elderly, on sun-exposed sites. It is the least malignant variety of melanoma, and is preceded by lentigo maligna (i.e. the *in situ* growth phase). It commonly presents as an irregular brown patch over the cheek, and malignant change is usually associated with the development of discrete, raised nodules within the lesion. Metastasis to lymph nodes is less common than for other malignant melanomas. Early intervention (e.g. by cryotherapy) during the lateral growth phase carries a good prognosis.

It is important to note that unlike lentigo maligna, amelanotic melanoma is non-pigmented; similarly, acral-lentiginous melanoma is more common in the extremities, palm, and sole. Acral lentiginous melanoma is mostly seen in Japanese people and in dark-skinned races. As with nodular melanomas, their prognosis is poor.

Finally, superficial spreading melanoma (i.e. the most common subtype in both sexes), usually presents at about 40 years of age. It is commonly seen on sun-exposed skin—women tend to be affected on the back of the lower leg, whilst men are affected in the upper back. It may arise *de novo* or in association with a pre-existing naevus, and grows radially before vertical invasion. Patients present with lesions that may be irregularly brown, black, or bluish black, frequently associated with inflammation. Active vertical invasion manifests clinically as raised and ulcerated nodules, and is a poor prognostic sign.

3. Keratoacanthoma is a rapidly growing epidermal tumour that resembles squamous cell carcinoma both clinically and histologically. It is believed to arise from hair follicles and is seen mostly on sun-exposed sites. It is usually presents as a single, fleshy, elevated, and nodular lesion with a central hyperkeratotic core. The most significant histological feature is its rapid growth rate. There is little evidence that this lesion has malignant potential, although it mimics the histological features of squamous cell carcinoma. Trauma, viruses, sun exposure, and chronic exposure to tar, pitch, and petroleum have been implicated as aetiological agents. Although spontaneous resolution tends to occur, surgical excision may product less scarring than the former. In this case, the short history and rapid increase in size suggest a diagnosis of keratoacanthoma rather than squamous cell carcinoma.

3. Answers: 1-G; 2-F; 3-I

1. The radial nerve arises from nerve roots C5–T1 of the brachial plexus and is an important nerve supplying the dorsal aspect of the arm and forearm. It supplies the triceps, brachioradialis, wrist extensors, and extensor digitorum longus muscles. The sensory supply of the radial nerve includes the dorsum of the thumb and the first dorsal web space, and the dorsum of the forearm. In any form of radial nerve injury, the clinical extent of the disability depends on the level of the lesion.

In this scenario, the patient has sustained a high radial nerve lesion (i.e. as occurs with fractures of the humerus — particularly mid-shaft fractures, where the radial nerve lies in the spiral grove; or after prolonged tourniquet pressure). In such cases, there may be weakness of the radial extensors of the wrist, and numbness over the anatomical snuffbox. Such patterns are also seen in patients who fall asleep with their arm dangling over the back of a chair (i.e. 'Saturday night palsy').

2. In this scenario, the patient is likely to have sustained a very high lesion of her radial nerve (i.e. at the level of the axilla). When the radial nerve is compressed in the axilla (e.g. during high-speed RTAs or from the inappropriate use of crutches, etc.), patients may experience complete paralysis of the triceps, paralysis of the extensors supplied by the radial nerve (thus resulting in wrist drop), and loss of the triceps reflex. Similarly, such a mechanism of injury results in sensory loss over the dorsum of the forearm, thumb and the first dorsal web space.

3. The ulnar nerve arises from the C8 and T1 nerve roots of the brachial plexus and is an important nerve of the upper limb. Laceration at the level of the wrist (i.e. usually from trauma) is the most common cause of low ulnar nerve lesions. Pressure from deep ganglia may also cause such symptoms. It is important to note that lesions of the ulnar nerve at the level of the wrist will produce hypothenar wasting and clawing of the hand due to the action of the unopposed long flexors.

As is described in this scenario, the sensory loss experienced in ulnar nerve lesions is confined to the skin over the little and ring fingers. Patients may experience notable difficulty with gripping (or pinching) objects since finger abduction and thumb adduction are lost. This results from paralysis of the adductor pollicis and the first palmar interossei, which results in flexion of the thumb due to the unopposed action of the flexor pollicis longus muscle. It can be demonstrated by asking the patient to grasp a card between the thumb and index finger, and noting the pronounced flexion at the interphalangeal joint of the thumb, instead of adduction at the metacarpophalangeal joint (i.e. Froment's sign).

4. Answers: 1-H; 2-F; 3-G

1. Pyrexia is a common postoperative finding after most types of surgery. The underlying cause of the pyrexia may be determined by its time of onset relative to surgery, the type of surgery that was performed, and the associated clinical findings. Low-grade pyrexia that occurs within the first 24 hours of surgery is commonly due to the systemic response to trauma, or due to pre-existing infection. The physiological systemic inflammatory response that occurs involves the release of inflammatory cytokines such as interferon (IL)-1, IL-2 and tumour necrosis factor. These cytokines act as pyrogens and their effects may manifest as soon as two hours after the initial incision.

2. Pyrexia that occurs within 24–72 hours of surgery may be attributed to pulmonary atelectasis or pneumonia. The patient in this scenario is not producing purulent sputum and has not developed a sufficiently raised temperature to suggest the presence of pneumonia. Chest radiography may demonstrate basal lung collapse with atelectasis, and the appearance of consolidation in pneumonia. Atelectasis, which is a common complication following thoraco-abdominal surgery and general anaesthesia, results from diaphragmatic splinting (i.e. insufficient respiratory excursion secondary to pain) and dysfunction of surfactant, causing the alveoli to collapse. Patients with atelectasis should be managed with adequate analgesia, nebulized saline and chest physiotherapy.

3. Deep venous thrombosis (DVT) and pulmonary embolism (PE) may present 7-10 days following surgery (i.e. especially operations resulting in a considerable degree of postoperative immobility, thereby encouraging venous stasis and thrombosis). The patient in this scenario is at high risk of venous thromboembolic disease, and demonstrates the signs and symptoms of a PE that originated as a DVT within the leg. In addition to tachycardia, tachypnoea and low-grade pyrexia, patients may experience pleuritic chest pain, dizziness or syncope. The diagnosis of PE is best confirmed by CTPA, or alternatively by ventilation/perfusion scanning of the lungs.

5. Answers: 1-H; 2-C; 3-B

1. Burns can be classified according to their depth. Superficial burns are painful, pink and dry, with brisk blanching and bleeding. Superficial partial-thickness burns appear pink and wet with fine blisters; they also blanch and bleed easily. Deep partial-thickness burns, however, are less painful but appear bright red and do not blanch. Full-thickness burns are dry, leathery, hairless, insensate, and do not blanch.

2. There are several ways to estimate the injured percentage of total body surface area for a patient with burns. These include:

- Wallace's Rule of Nines: This arbitrarily divides the body into units of surface area divisible by nine (with the exception of the perineum). In an adult, the respective percentages of the total body surface area are approximately 9% for the head and neck (i.e. front and back); 9% for each upper limb (i.e. front and back); 18% for the front of the thorax and abdomen; 18% for the back of the thorax and abdomen; 1% for the perineum; and 18% for each lower limb (i.e. front and back). This system is relatively accurate for adults but not for children, due to their relatively disproportionate body part surface area. In this scenario, the patient's burnt back (18%), arm (9%) and thigh (9%) comprise 36% of the total body surface area.
- Lund and Browder chart: this chart provides the most accurate method for estimating burn extent, and must be used in the evaluation of paediatric patients with burns.
- Palmar surface area: the patient's palm is deemed equivalent to 1% of his/her total body surface area.

3. The Muir and Barclay formula calculates the volume of fluid (i.e. colloid resuscitation with plasma) that needs to be administered in addition to maintenance fluid, over the initial 36-hour period.

Replacement fluid volume (mL) = [body weight (kg) × burn surface area (%)] / 2

For this patient, replacement volume = [65 × 36]/2= 1170 mL. This volume of fluid should be given 4-, 4-, 4-, 6-, 6-, and 12-hourly. Therefore, for the first 12 hours, the volume required is 1170 × 3 = 3510 mL.

It is also important to understand the Parkland formula for fluid resuscitation for burns, which is used by certain specialist burns centres. By the Parkland formula, fluid requirements (e.g. crystalloid resuscitation with Hartmann's solution) for the first 24 hours are:

Replacement fluid volume (mL) = 4 × body weight (kg) × burn surface area (%)

Half of this volume is given in the first 8 hours from the time of the burn, while the remaining volume is given in the next 16 hours. In addition, patients need maintenance fluid in addition to resuscitation fluid to replace any potential evaporative losses and metabolic requirements. In a fit adult, this usually involves 2–2.5 L (of normal saline with potassium) daily. It is vital that this volume is modified according to the likely physiological reserves of the patient, through careful clinical and biochemical monitoring.

6. Answers: 1-H; 2-G; 3-D

1. *Pseudomonas aeruginosa* is a Gram-negative bacillus. It causes infection in immunocompromised patients (e.g. bronchopneumonia in patients with cystic fibrosis and necrotizing enterocolitis in premature infants and neutropaenic patients) by releasing exotoxins. It also causes skin and soft tissue haemorrhage and necrosis in burns victims and in neutropaenic sepsis.

2. Staghorn calculi (i.e. 'struvite', comprising magnesium ammonium phosphate) are invariably associated with urinary tract infections—specifically, the presence of urease-producing bacteria, such as *Proteus mirabilis*. This results in the hydrolysis of urea into ammonia and hydroxyl ions. The ammonia and the phosphate ions subsequently combine with the alkalotic urine environment, resulting in struvite and carbonate apatite crystallization.

3. *Clostridium perfringens* infection results from the inoculation of the organism within tissue of low oxygen tension. The organisms then multiply and produce exotoxins, which results in myonecrosis. More than half of such cases are preceded by trauma, compound fractures, amputations, abortions and gastrointestinal surgery. They may present with oedema, erythema, skin discoloration, extreme tenderness, skin crepitations, and a profuse, non-purulent and thin serous discharge from ruptured bullae.

7. Answers: 1-B; 2-E; 3-A

1. This patient's pathology is classified as Dukes' A colorectal carcinoma. As the patient has already undergone surgery (i.e. the definitive, curative treatment for early colorectal cancer) and is now known to have no tumour-positive lymph nodes or distant metastasis, he may simply be managed with surveillance as dictated by local protocol.

2. This patient's pathology is classified as Dukes' C colorectal carcinoma. In such cases, adjuvant chemotherapy with 5-fluorouracil (5-FU) and leucovorin (folinic acid) reduces the incidence of recurrence by approximately 41%. In stage III colon cancer, the addition of oxaliplatin with 5-FU and leucovorin as adjuvant therapy is associated with a 24% reduction in the relative risk of cancer recurrence after 3 years, when compared to chemotherapy involving 5-FU and leucovorin alone.

3. As this elderly patient has been found to have distant metastasis, palliative therapy and supportive care is the most appropriate treatment option. For patients with metastatic colorectal cancer who are deemed fit for (and who are agreeable to) palliative chemotherapy, trials of 5-FU and leucovorin have demonstrated improved response rates, improved quality of life, and better survival when compared with single-agent 5-FU therapies. Other chemotherapeutic agents used in metastatic colorectal cancer include oxaliplatin, irinotecan and bevacizumab.

8. Answers: 1-G; 2-B; 3-H

1. Enteral nutrition is the best route for nutritional support since it reduces the incidence of peptic ulceration, decreases liver and renal dysfunction, decreases bacterial translocation from the gut, and reduces the incidence of feeding line and other stoma-related complications. Since this patient is recovering from a head injury (and was previously fit and healthy), nasoenteric fine-bore feeding is an appropriate method of nutritional support since it is likely that he will recover sufficiently within a few days to take food and drink orally.

2. It is not possible or appropriate to institute or provide enteral nutrition in certain patients (e.g. patients with short bowel syndrome, or after oesophagectomy or gastrectomy). PEG is the preferred method to feed patients who are unable to eat or swallow food due to debilitating conditions such as stroke or cancer, in whom long-term nutritional support is indicated. It also decompresses the stomach over a prolonged period of time.

3. This patient is undergoing a Lewis–Tanner procedure where the affected segment of the oesophagus, along with the tumour and the surrounding perioesophageal tissue with adjacent lymph nodes, are resected. This procedure is undertaken through a right-sided thoracotomy along with a laparotomy. A perioperative jejunostomy is usually fashioned to feed these patients postoperatively.

9. Answers: 1-H; 2-A; 3-D

1. The Kruskal–Wallis test is a non-parametric test that is used when there are more than two groups to compare. The formula is based on the ranks of the scores, rather than the scores themselves. The test is used to look for a significant difference between the mean ranks of some or all of the conditions.

2. A correlation coefficient is a number between '−1' and '+1', which measures the degree to which two variables are linearly related. A correlation coefficient of '0' means that there is no linear relationship between the variables. The Spearman rank correlation coefficient is used in non-parametric studies and is usually calculated on occasions when it is not convenient or possible to give actual values to variables, but only to assign a rank order to instances of each variable. It is a better indicator to suggest that a relationship exists between two variables when the relationship is non-linear.

3. In clinical trials, the time until participants in a particular study present specific events or end-point is often a crucial point of interest. This event is usually a clinical outcome and the time can be described using the Kaplan–Meier curve.

10. Answers: 1-D; 2-F; 3-H

1. This patient has a pelvic abscess. Pelvic abscesses can occur following abdominal surgeries or gynaecological interventions such as medical termination of pregnancy. It can present either in the first few days following the procedure or up to 2–3 weeks later. The signs and symptoms are

typical of any intraperitoneal abscess such as swinging pyrexia, chills and rigors, and malaise. Per rectal examination reveals tenderness in the pelvic region. Blood inflammatory markers such as white cell count (WCC), ESR, or C-reactive protein (CRP) may be elevated. The diagnosis is confirmed with a pelvic USS.

2. Upper urinary tract infection in combination with obstruction and hydronephrosis may lead to pyonephrosis. It may develop from a broad spectrum of pathological conditions involving either an ascending infection of the urinary tract or the haematogenous spread of a bacterial pathogen. Common clinical features include pyrexia, rigors, and pain in the affected loin. However, some patients may be asymptomatic initially whilst others may present with frank sepsis. A mass (hydronephrosis) may be felt in the loin region. Diabetes mellitus is a recognized risk factor for developing pyonephrosis.

3. Subphrenic abscesses usually arise as a result of direct contamination after surgery especially of the biliary tract, duodenum or stomach, or a perforated viscus. The other causes include infections or trauma to the liver and gall bladder. The subphrenic space is in direct contact with the paracolic gutter, thereby allowing peritoneal contamination such as bile, blood, or bowel contents to spread. Clinical features include pyrexia, anorexia, loss of appetite, and loss of weight. Diaphragmatic irritation may affect the lung which may result in chest pain, dyspnoea, and non-productive cough. Basal atelectasis, pneumonia, and pleural effusion are also recognized complications which cause percussion dullness and decreased breath sounds on the affected side.

11. Answers: 1-A; 2-B; 3-C

1. The signs and symptoms in this patient are suggestive of a HAP. HAP develops at least 48 hours after hospital admission. Postoperative pneumonia develops usually 36–72 hours following surgery. Common organisms causing HAP include *Streptococcus pneumoniae*, *Haemophilus influenzae*, *Staphylococcus aureus*, and Gram-negative bacteria. Ventilator-associated pneumonia (VAP) is defined as pneumonia developing at least 48 hours after mechanical ventilation.

2. The signs and symptoms in this patient are suggestive of a PE. PE occurs in 50% of patients with DVT. They can be non-massive (<50% obstruction), massive (>50% obstruction), or multiple minor PEs. Massive PE causes haemodynamic instability by causing obstruction of the flow of blood to the left atrium. PE usually presents with dyspnoea, and pleuritic chest pain. Sinus tachycardia is the commonest ECG abnormality associated with PE (the classical '$S_IQ_{III}T_{III}$' pattern is rarely seen). Arterial blood gases show hypoxaemia, hypocapnoea, and respiratory alkalosis due to hyperventilation.

3. The presence of ischaemic heart disease in an elderly patient with the described signs and symptoms is highly suggestive of pulmonary oedema. Acute pulmonary oedema is characterized by acute breathlessness, anxiety, tachycardia, sweating, and cardiogenic shock in severe cases. Signs include fine crepitations in the lung bases and a raised jugular venous pressure (JVP). Treatment includes high-flow oxygen, intravenous furosemide, diamorphine, sublingual glyceryl trinitrate (GTN) ± GTN infusion.

12. Answers: 1-B; 2-C; 3-B; 4-D

1. There are some circumstances in which patients under the Mental Health Act 1983 can have only their mental disorder treated without their consent. It does not apply to any physical disorders, for which the usual consent applies. This patient is being treated compulsorily for her mental illness under the Mental Health Act and is therefore unable to give an informed consent.

In this situation, as the surgeon and the psychiatrist agree that surgery in the best treatment option, the surgeon can proceed with the laparotomy.

2. Competent adults may refuse treatment. A competent pregnant woman may refuse treatment even if detrimental to the fetus. Nobody can give or refuse treatment on their behalf.

3. Incompetent adults must be treated in their best interests; this may not equate to best medical interests. Nobody can give or refuse consent on their behalf. The professional judgement should stand up to the Bolam test (reasonable body of medical opinion). Advance care directives and legal wills are legally binding and should be followed.

4. Children under 16 or those that are 16–17 years old, but incompetent, generally need a parent or guardian to give consent. Refusal of treatment by the parents of a child which is deemed in the child's best interests may need a second opinion and referral to the courts.

13. Answers: 1-C; 2-E; 3-B

1. Intracapsular fractures of the femoral neck (i.e. as opposed to extracapsular fractures) risk avascular necrosis of the femoral head due to disruption of the retinacular vessels and the nutrient artery. They rely primarily on the artery within the ligamentum teres, which cannot usually perfuse the femoral head independently. Intracapsular fractures can be classified as per the Garden classification, based on plain anteroposterior radiography of the hip. In this scenario, the fracture is intertrochanteric and therefore extracapsular in nature.

Dynamic hip screws can be used for inter trochanteric fractures to allow gradual collapse of the femoral head. It is not used in intracapsular fractures as the head would spin around the axis of the screw and damage the blood supply. This is the quickest and easiest operation which can be performed in the elderly patient presenting with this type of fracture, to return them back to their premorbid state of function.

2. Radiography of the hip in this scenario demonstrates the most severe of intracapsular fractures of the femoral neck (i.e. a Garden type IV fracture), where complete fracturing and full displacement is evident. The most suitable course of action is hemiarthroplasty of the hip with an Austin Moore prosthesis, which is the treatment of choice for elderly (>70 years) patients with comorbidities, presenting with Garden type III or IV fractures. It is used in patients who already have poor mobility and are at a lower risk of acetabular damage from the new hip prosthesis.

3. The radiographic findings of this patient's hip are consistent with a Garden type II fracture (i.e. a complete or 'bicortical' fracture with no displacement). In patients with Garden type I or II fractures, cannulated hip screws are widely regarded as the treatment of choice. Internal fixation may be performed with three cannulated hip screws to prevent the head spinning around an axis, thereby also preserving the joint. It should be noted that some surgeons also elect to use cannulated screws as an initial measure for the more severe Garden type III and IV fractures in young (i.e. aged <60 years) patients.

14. Answers: 1-E; 2-B; 3-F

1. Curative surgery for ulcerative colitis historically entailed panproctocolectomy with ileostomy formation. However, a more recent alternative (i.e. restorative proctocolectomy) has largely avoided the need for a permanent stoma. This procedure is performed in two stages: firstly, a proctocolectomy is performed while preserving the anus and anal sphincter. An ileal pouch is then fashioned and anastomosed with the anus. A temporary loop ileostomy is also formed, to allow the distal anastomosis to heal over 8–10 weeks. At this point, the ileostomy is reversed

and patients can expect to have an average of six bowel movements per day (of mostly soft stool). Patients should be well motivated and prepared to deal with potential complications of this procedure, which include pouchitis (30%, managed with antibiotics such as metronidazole or ciprofloxacin); bowel obstruction (secondary to adhesions and usually managed conservatively); anastomotic leakage, and pouch failure (which requires pouch removal and conversion to a permanent ileostomy).

2. Unlike small bowel obstruction, which most commonly results from adhesions and hernias, large bowel obstruction is caused primarily by colorectal malignancy. This diagnosis is largely supported by the patient's age and radiographic findings, although the presenting history may reveal more features suggestive of progressive malignancy. The operation of choice for an obstructing sigmoid tumour is a Hartmann's procedure. A sigmoid colectomy is performed, with the proximal segment exteriorized as a colostomy, and the distal segment closed off and left *in situ*. Primary anastomosis should be avoided due to the higher risk of anastomotic leak in patients presenting with bowel obstruction.

3. The primary procedure in this scenario is a sigmoid colectomy, thus removing the tumour. If no evidence of perforation was noted intraoperatively, a primary anastomosis may have been performed. However, the presence of faecal peritonitis greatly increases the chance of contamination and subsequent anastomotic leakage in the early postoperative period. For similar reasons, the distal stump of a Hartmann's procedure is also at risk after faecal peritonitis. A mucus fistula is therefore fashioned by exteriorizing the distal segment, allowing mucus secretions to drain from the distal colon. This may subsequently be reversed and re-anastomosis performed within 4–8 weeks after the primary procedure.

15. Answers: 1-A; 2-D; 3-E

1. Aminoglycoside antibiotics include amikacin, gentamycin, neomycin, streptomycin, etc. They can be bacteriocidal or bacteriostatic depending on the dosages administered. They are active against Gram-negative and Gram-positive organisms. They are primarily excreted via the kidneys and therefore their accumulation occurs in renal impairment. Due to renal excretion, gentamycin is an effective antibiotic in the treatment of pyelonephritis. Most side effects are dose-related, therefore any dosages should be carefully calculated according to the patient's weight, and treatment should not exceed 7 days.

2. Cephalosporins are grouped into first-, second-, third-, and fourth-generation cephalosporins depending on their antimicrobial properties. Each subsequent generation has a greater Gram-negative antimicrobial effect against resistance than the previous. Cefuroxime is the commonest cephalosporin used in surgical prophylaxis and in the treatment of biliary sepsis, diverticulitis and faecal peritonitis. Their most common side effect is hypersensitivity and about 10% of penicillin-allergic patients will also be allergic to cephalosporins.

3. Fluoroquinolones are broad-spectrum antibiotics that are considered to be synthetic chemotherapeutic agents as they exert their antimicrobial effects by interfering with DNA synthesis. Ofloxacin, ciprofloxacin, and moxifloxacin are a few examples of such drugs. They readily cross the placenta and are secreted in breast milk, thereby predisposing to birth defects and miscarriage; they are therefore contraindicated in pregnancy. The toxicity of some drugs metabolized by cytochrome P450 is enhanced by the use of some quinolones, e.g. when used with warfarin, the international normalized ratio (INR) may dangerously rise. Ciprofloxacin may also reduce phenytoin plasma levels and reduce seizure threshold in susceptible patients.

16. Answers: 1-F; 2-B; 3-C

1. The presence of hypercoagulable states such as factor V Leiden mutation, protein C and protein S deficiency, and antiphospholipid syndrome, is an indication to institute aggressive prophylaxis against thromboembolic disease. This should include high-dose prophylactic low-molecular-weight heparin, pneumatic compression stockings, and early postoperative mobilization. This should be continued until the day of discharge. However, recent evidence suggests that the coagulation cascade is persistently active up to 4 weeks after surgical intervention and high-risk patients may therefore benefit from thromboprophylaxis during this time.

2. A history of upper gastrointestinal bleeding and major surgery are both contraindications for anticoagulation in this patient. However, he is at high risk of propagating his DVT and developing further thrombosis due to risk factors such as malignancy, chemotherapy, major surgery, and immobilization. Inferior vena cava filters are indicated in such high-risk patients in whom anticoagulation is contraindicated.

3. In consideration of this patient's multiple PEs and other risk factors, it is vital to exclude the presence of concurrent DVT. Despite the fact that no aggressive treatment is likely to be required for his multiple (and likely chronic) small PEs, his major pelvic surgery risks the embolization of any pre-existing DVTs, significantly increasing the risk of perioperative mortality and morbidity. If the venous duplex USS confirms the presence of a DVT, the insertion of a vena cava filter may be considered to prevent such a complication.

17. Answers: 1-F; 2-C; 3-G

1. Acute closed-angle glaucoma is an ophthalmological emergency and normally occurs in older patients. The outflow of aqueous fluid is acutely interrupted at the peripheral iris, leading to an acute increase in intraocular pressure. Systemic symptoms include ocular pain, nausea, and vomiting. The eye is red with a hazy cornea and mid-dilated, oval pupil. Visual acuity is usually decreased. Urgent ophthalmological referral is key to managing this condition but if this cannot happen immediately, reduction of intra-ocular pressure by reducing aqueous secretion (e.g. with acetazolamide) and inducing pupillary constriction (e.g. with pilocarpine) may be warranted. Definitive management involves the use of drugs (e.g. miotics), laser iridoplasty, or surgical (or laser) iridectomy.

2. Scleritis refers to the inflammation of the sclera in the anterior/posterior segments of the eye and is uncommon. Over 50% of scleritis is caused by an underlying systemic condition such as rheumatoid arthritis, with 50% of cases being bilateral. Symptoms include a gradual increase in eye pain, which may become severe with tenderness on palpation. There is diffuse or sectoral tenderness, increased watering, and photophobia. Nodules may be present and complications include scleral thinning and corneal ulceration. Early ophthalmological referral is key in managing this condition. The condition itself is generally resistant to treatment, and systemic NSAIDs are commonly used for symptomatic relief.

3. Anterior uveitis refers to the inflammation of the anterior part of the uveal tract. It accounts for 75% of all cases of uveitis. It is usually unilateral and presents with pain, photophobia, circumlimbal injection, an irregular-shaped pupil and blurred vision. It is associated with systemic conditions like diabetes and sarcoidosis. Management involves systemic analgesics to relieve pain, dark glasses for photophobia, and dilation of the pupils (e.g. with mydiatric or cycloplegic agents) to prevent inflammatory adhesions. Whilst infectious causes of uveitis are treated with appropriate antiviral or antimicrobial agents, non-infectious causes are addressed with topical or systemic corticosteroids.

18. Answers: 1-B; 2-A; 3-F

1. Wounds that are otherwise clean and created during emergency surgery, e.g. right hemicolectomy or cholecystectomy, are considered to be 'clean contaminated' wounds. These have an infection rate of <10% and this risk is similar to patients who have reoperations via a clean incision within 7 days, where there is minor break in aseptic technique or where the viscus is opened but no spillage of gut contents occur.

2. Elective procedures such as mastectomy and hernia repairs are classified as clean procedures as they involve incisions that are made through non-inflamed tissue. The wounds are primarily closed and only closed drainage systems are used. This risk increases if a hollow viscus is accidentally opened.

3. In the presence of pus in the form of an intraperitoneal abscess or visceral perforation, any surgery is classified as dirty and the patient therefore has a 40% risk of developing a wound infection. This is a similar risk as wound infection from penetrating trauma of over 4 hours' duration.

19. Answers: 1-E; 2-G; 3-C

1. The diagnosis of fat embolism syndrome (FES) is based on the Gurd and Wilson criteria. One major criterion, four minor criteria, and the presence of fat macroglobulinaemia is required for the diagnosis of FES. The major criteria include petechial rash on the upper body, respiratory symptoms and signs or changes on chest radiography, and cerebral signs unrelated to head injury. Minor criteria include tachycardia, pyrexia, retinal changes, renal changes and jaundice. In addition to fat macroglobulinaemia, other laboratory indicators include a drop in haemoglobin, sudden thrombocytopenia, and high ESR. Treatment of this patient should involve reduction and immobilization of the fracture as well as support of respiratory, cardiovascular, and central nervous systems.

2. Embolization of a thrombus in new-onset atrial fibrillation and end-organ hypoperfusion from cardiac failure are the commonest causes of gut ischaemia. The atrophic gut mucosa allows bacterial translocation and a resultant systemic inflammatory response. The cytokine-led endothelial damage results in vasodilatation and extravasation of fluid into the interstitial spaces resulting in hypotension and tachycardia. The circulating endotoxins also have a direct inflammatory effect, resulting in myocardial dysfunction. The kidneys are presented with inflammatory matter to filter and hypoperfusion which leads to an elevated urea and creatinine. Multiorgan dysfunction syndrome refers to the progression from SIRS resulting in end-organ dysfunction. It is diagnosed by dysfunction of two or more organ systems (gastrointestinal tract, renal and cardiovascular functions in this patient).

3. Acute respiratory distress syndrome (ARDS) refers to the pulmonary component of SIRS and is characterized by the acute onset of respiratory symptoms, hypoxia refractory to oxygen therapy, new bilateral pulmonary infiltrates on chest radiography, a pulmonary artery wedge pressure of <18 mmHg and a $PaO_2:FiO_2$ ratio of <200 mmHg. These patients often require mechanical ventilation. Their airway pressures remain high during positive pressure ventilation due to poor lung compliance. Smoke inhalation results in the activation of neutrophils and the release of inflammatory mediators, which cause direct capillary endothelial cell damage and protein-rich exudates from the alveoli.

20. Answers: 1-A; 2-B; 3-J

1. *Staphylococcus aureus* is a Gram-positive coccus. It is commonly found in the nose and skin. Diseases caused by the bacteria range from simple skin infections to severe pneumonia and sepsis. The bacteria produce toxins which lead to the various spectrum of disease.

2. *Enterococcus* is a genus of lactic acid bacteria. They are Gram-positive cocci often occurring in pairs. Common commensal organisms include *E. faecalis* and *E. faecium*. Important infections caused by *Enterococcus* species include diverticulitis, bacterial endocarditis, urinary tract infections, and meningitis. They demonstrate a high level of intrinsic antibiotic resistance; particularly virulent strains that are resistant to vancomycin have emerged in the tertiary care setting.

3. Normal stool contains over 500 types of bacteria. When antibiotics suppress drug-sensitive organisms within normal gut flora, *C. difficile* is allowed to multiply and produce exotoxins A and B. Exotoxin A is an enterotoxin that causes increased secretions from the gastrointestinal tract, resulting in watery diarrhoea. Exotoxin B is a cytotoxin that causes damage to the colonic mucosa, leading to pseudomembrane formation. The diagnosis of C. difficile pseudomembranous colitis is confirmed by the detection of toxin by enzyme-linked immunosorbent assay (ELISA) of infected stool samples. It should be noted that 10% of patients on broad-spectrum antibiotics develop diarrhoea, and 1% of patients will develop pseudomembranous colitis.

21. Answers: 1-E; 2-C; 3-D; 4-H

The considerations towards adjuvant chemotherapy for malignant disease of the breast are based on the risk of recurrence and hormone receptor status of the tumour; as well as the age, menopausal status and fitness of the patient. Patients who are under the age of 40 who have large, undifferentiated or poorly differentiated ER-negative tumours, or involved nodes, are the most likely individuals to benefit from chemotherapy.

Adjuvant radiotherapy is indicated following breast conservation surgery for invasive tumours or high-grade DCIS. It is recommended following mastectomy for patients at high risk of local recurrence (i.e. with tumours of large size or high grade; or tumours that are node positive or demonstrate evidence of vascular invasion).

Adjuvant hormone therapy is suitable for patients with ER-positive tumours for a period of 5 years. Oestrogen receptor antagonists (e.g. tamoxifen) may be used in women before or after menopause, while aromatase inhibitors (e.g. anastrozole, letrozole) are used in postmenopausal women.

Neoadjuvant chemotherapy is used to downstage locally advanced but non-metastatic cancer in patients who prefer breast conservation surgery to mastectomy. Approximately 40–50% of tumours are downstaged sufficiently. However, there is currently no evidence from prospective randomized control trials to suggest that neoadjuvant chemotherapy improves survival. The other indication for neoadjuvant chemotherapy is inflammatory breast cancer.

Neoadjuvant hormone therapy is used in a similar manner. Elderly patients with large, ER-positive tumours may benefit from initial hormone therapy using aromatase inhibitors prior to surgery.

Aromatase inhibitors may also harbour benefit for elderly patients in whom surgery and chemotherapy may not be appropriate forms of management.

1. The young age and advanced nature of this woman's tumour would prompt an aggressive approach (e.g. with adjuvant radiotherapy, chemotherapy and tamoxifen) after mastectomy and axillary clearance.

2. The advanced age and multiple comorbidities of this patient would put her at high risk for any form of aggressive therapy. Lifelong hormonal therapy with an aromatase inhibitor (e.g. letrozole) would therefore be most appropriate for this patient.

3. Although this patient is similar in age to the patient in Question 1 (above), the less advanced characteristics of her tumour implies that she is likely to benefit from adjuvant radiotherapy and tamixofen alone, with periodic follow-up scheduled thereafter.

4. The low-grade DCIS demonstrated on histology of this young patient's ER-positive tumour offers an even better prognosis to those of the patients in Questions 1 and 3 (above), and implies that she is likely to benefit from a 5-year regimen of tamoxifen treatment alone.

22. Answers: 1-I; 2-F; 3-G

1. Vicryl® or polyglactin is a braided, multifilament, synthetic suture that provides wound support for only 30 days. It elicits minimal tissue reaction and is absorbed by hydrolysis between 56–70 days. It is the most commonly used absorbable suture in general surgery as it handles well (with secure knot structure) due to its braid. A more rapidly absorbable form called Vicryl Rapide® is also available.

2. Prolene® or polypropylene is a synthetic, non-absorbable monofilament which slides easily, making it the suture of choice for vascular anastomosis. However, this characteristic makes it difficult to knot and more challenging to handle as it has a significant memory. Another disadvantage is that inadvertent crushing of the suture can result in a 90% loss in tensile strength and therefore great care needs to be taken during vascular anastomosis.

3. Silk is a natural, braided or twisted multifilament suture that is non-absorbable. It undergoes fibrous encapsulation in the body after 2–3 weeks and has a high incidence of tissue reaction as it lingers on for 1–2 years before it slowly degrades. Infection can linger in its braided structure and encourage the formation of suture sinuses and abscesses. Due to such properties, it is no longer used routinely in surgical practice, apart from securing drains in place.

23. Answers: 1-E; 2-C; 3-I

1. When there is an extended time period during two courses of radiotherapy, a proportion of surviving cells are able to undergo mitosis, thereby increasing the total number of malignant cells that need to be killed during the course of radiotherapy. Evidence has demonstrated that the control of head and neck cancers has improved considerably by shortening the overall treatment time. This benefit has also been observed in the treatment of lung cancers with CHART.

2. These sources of sealed radiotherapy can be removed once the treatment is complete. Some examples of the use of this modality of radiotherapy include the use of caesium for the treatment of cervical cancer and the use of iridium in the treatment of anal, and head and neck malignancies.

3. Radioactive iodine can be used in patients following surgical resection of anaplastic, papillary, or follicular tumours of the thyroid, in order to ablate the residual tumour cells in the thyroid or those which have metastasized to lymph nodes. These agents have a relatively short half-life of about 8 days, and relatively low radiation emission in order to protect the surrounding tissue from radiation damage.

24. Answers: 1-C; 2-D; 3-H

1. Ethylene oxide is a hazardous organic compound. At room temperature it is flammable, carcinogenic, and an irritant. It inhibits the growth of micro-organisms and can completely destroy

them by inducing the clotting of proteins and deactivation of enzymes. It works well at destroying Gram-positive bacteria and less so against fungi.

2. An autoclave is an instrument used to sterilize equipment. It uses steam at high pressures and high temperatures. The procedure lasts for 15–20 minutes and is used not only for sterilizing equipment for re-use but also for predisposal treatment of waste material. The process destroys all bacteria, viruses, spores, and fungi but not prions. Heat-sensitive equipment cannot be sterilized with this procedure.

3. The use of sporicidal chemicals is another effective means of sterilization. Bacterial spores are very resistant to biocides, and sporicidal effectiveness is largely dependent on which part of the cell cycle the spore is at. The compounds employed for this procedure are often toxic and an irritant. 2% glutaraldehyde is the most widely used liquid sporicidal chemical, and can effectively eliminate viruses and bacteria within 10 minutes.

1. Common surgical conditions and the subspecialties: Gastrointestinal disease

A. Ischaemic colitis
B. Angiodysplasia
C. Ulcerative colitis
D. Blind loop syndrome
E. Fulminating colitis
F. Diverticulitis
G. Crohn's disease
H. Intestinal obstruction
I. Carcinoma of the rectum

For each of the following situations, select the single most likely diagnosis from the options listed. Each option may be used once, more than once, or not at all.

1. A 44-year-old lady presents to the surgical outpatient clinic with a 4-month history of increased frequency of bowel motions (i.e. up to 10 times daily). The stools are associated with blood and mucus. She has lost 15 kg in weight during this period. Rigid sigmoidoscopy reveals an inflamed sigmoid colon and a number of small ulcers in the rectum.

2. A 66-year-old man, known to have inflammatory bowel disease, is brought to the Emergency Department with severe abdominal pain. On examination, he appears pale and dehydrated, and is febrile with a temperature of 37.7°C and a tachycardia of 110/min. He has generalized abdominal tenderness and guarding. Plain abdominal radiography reveals grossly dilated large bowel, with a maximum wall-to-wall diameter of 6 cm (transverse colon).

3. A 77-year-old woman is brought to the Emergency Department with a 3-hour history of severe, colicky abdominal pain and vomiting. Her blood pressure is 90/70 mmHg and her pulse rate is 112/min, with an irregularly irregular rhythm. Abdominal examination reveals evidence of peritonism. Whilst in the Emergency Department, she also passes bright red blood per rectum.

2. **Common surgical conditions and the subspecialties: Trauma and orthopaedics**

   A. Bunion
   B. Bursitis
   C. Capsulitis
   D. Fibroma
   E. Ingrowing toenail
   F. March fracture
   G. Morton's neuroma
   H. Paronychia
   I. Tarsal tunnel syndrome
   J. Synovial sarcoma

   For each of the following situations, select the single most likely diagnosis from the options listed. Each option may be used once, more than once, or not at all.

   1. A 48-year-old secretary presents to her GP with a 3-month history of intermittent, sharp pain in her forefoot at work, associated with occasional numbness and burning of her 3rd and 4th toes. The pain is relieved by removing her shoes and massaging the affected region. Examination reveals decreased sensation between the 3rd and 4th toes.

   2. A 35-year-old cleaner presents to her GP with a 2-month history of progressively worsening, dull ache and stiffness in her left big toe. The pain is exacerbated by movement at the interphalangeal joint and relieved by simple analgesia. Examination reveals tenderness at the affected interphalangeal joint and warmth over the surrounding skin.

   3. A 41-year-old mountaineer presents to his GP with an 18-month history of progressive lancinating pain in his left foot radiating directly from the ankle to the bottom of the foot arch. His symptoms are worsened by prolonged walking and standing. Examination reveals normal foot pulses but the patient's symptoms are reproduced with passive pronation of the foot.

3. **The assessment and management of the surgical patient:
   Surgical history and examination**

   A. Common peroneal nerve
   B. Deep peroneal nerve
   C. Lateral cutaneous nerve of thigh
   D. Lateral plantar nerve
   E. Medial plantar nerve
   F. Saphenous nerve
   G. Sciatic nerve
   H. Superficial peroneal nerve
   I. Sural nerve
   J. Tibial nerve

   For each of the following situations, select the single most likely nerve to be involved from the options listed. Each option may be used once, more than once, or not at all.

   1. A 28-year-old professional footballer is seen in the Emergency Department after sustaining an injury to his left leg from an aggressive tackle. During physical examination, he is unable to dorsiflex his left foot and demonstrates reduced sensation over the dorsum of his foot. Plain radiography demonstrates a fracture of the left fibular neck.

   2. A 36-year-old lady who is 34 weeks pregnant presents to her obstetrician with a 1-week history of pain and paraesthesia over the upper outer aspect of her right thigh. Her pregnancy has otherwise been uneventful. On examination, the patient demonstrates normal gait and there is no restriction of movements in her hips or knees.

   3. A 63-year-old secretary is referred by her GP to the orthopaedic outpatient clinic for a 3-day history of right foot drop and decreased sensation on the lateral side of her right leg below the knee. Her past medical history includes well-controlled asthma and diabetes mellitus, and a right total hip replacement 3 weeks prior to this.

4. Perioperative care: Postoperative complications

A. Acute bowel ischaemia
B. Acute gastric dilatation
C. Adynamic bowel obstruction
D. Anastomotic leak and abscess formation
E. Enterocutaneous fistula
F. Early postoperative ileus
G. Mechanical obstruction
H. Pseudo-obstruction
I. Systemic sepsis

For each of the following situations, select the single most likely postoperative complication from the options listed. Each option may be used once, more than once, or not at all.

1. A 55-year-old lady who has had multiple previous gynaecological operations is admitted with abdominal pain, distension and vomiting. She undergoes a laparotomy for division of adhesions and release of small bowel obstruction. The operation proves challenging and multiple peritoneal and omental windows have to be made by the surgical registrar. Two days after her operation, she still complains of abdominal pain and vomiting. On examination, her abdomen is distended and tympanic, with hyperactive bowel sounds. Plain abdominal radiography demonstrates distended loops of small bowel and distally collapsed large bowel.

2. A 75-year-old male undergoes an anterior resection for a sigmoid tumour. By postoperative day 7, his recovery is still sub-optimal. He feels lethargic and is complaining of vague lower abdominal discomfort. His vital signs reveal a swinging pyrexia and tachycardia. On examination, his abdomen is soft but tender in the left iliac fossa. His bowel sounds are reduced and a digital rectal examination reveals a tender, boggy swelling anteriorly.

3. A 27-year-old male with recurrent episodes of right iliac fossa pain and leucocytosis undergoes an open appendectomy. Intraoperatively, the appendix does not look inflamed. His postoperative stay is prolonged due to a wound infection for which he is receiving intravenous antibiotics. His appetite remains poor and he is not tolerating solid food well. On postoperative day 4, the surgeon notices a purulent discharge from a broken-down wound; and the presence of gas bubbles in the wound as the patient coughs.

5. **Assessment and management of patients with trauma (including the multiply injured patient): Assessment, scoring, and triage of adults and children**

   A. Aortic dissection
   B. Cardiac tamponade
   C. Diaphragmatic rupture
   D. Flail chest
   E. Massive haemothorax
   F. Oesophageal rupture
   G. Rib fracture
   H. Open pneumothorax
   I. Tension pneumothorax
   J. Tracheobronchial injury

   For each of the following situations, select the single most likely diagnosis from the options listed. Each option may be used once, more than once, or not at all.

   1. A 32-year-old male is involved in a high-speed deceleration collision. On arrival in the Emergency Department he exhibits evidence of stridor, tracheal deviation, and surgical emphysema in the neck. The Advanced Trauma Life Support (ATLS®) protocol is followed and a chest drain is inserted to relieve a right-sided pneumothorax. The patient does not show improvement following this but continues to leak air from the chest drain.

   2. A 25-year-old prisoner presents to the Emergency Department 36 hours after being punched in the face, neck, and chest by his fellow inmates. Whilst awaiting further assessment, he complains of severe pain in the neck and chest, odynophagia and dysphonia. Examination reveals tachycardia, tachypnoea and subcutaneous emphysema of the patient's neck and chest.

   3. A 50-year-old male is brought to the Emergency Department after having been involved in a road traffic accident. His initial assessment reveals no evidence of external injury or blood loss. However, he subsequently complains of severe tearing pain in his back and hoarseness of voice. A senior review is requested, and on repeat examination, the patient is found to have a pulse rate of 140/min and respiratory rate of 27/min; and a 30 mmHg difference in blood pressure is noted between both of his arms.

6.   **Basic and applied sciences: Pharmacology**

A. Alkylating agents

B. Anti-tumour antibiotics

C. Antimetabolites

D. Antimicrotubule agents

E. Enzymes

F. Plant alkaloids

G. Retinoids

H. Ribonucleotide reductase inhibitors

I. Topoisomerase inhibitors

For each of the following descriptions, select the single most appropriate category of drugs from the options listed. Each option may be used once, more than once, or not at all.

1.   These chemotherapeutic agents act by adding a specific molecular group to the guanine base of tumour cell DNA, causing DNA damage and cell death. They are most active during the resting phase of the cell cycle. Some examples of these agents include cyclophosphamide, melphalan and chlorambucil.

2.   These chemotherapeutic agents act by becoming incorporated into the cellular metabolism and arresting cell growth and division at various stages of the cell cycle. They may be classified into antifolate drugs, purine analogues, pyrimidine analogues and adenosine deaminase inhibitors.

3.   These chemotherapeutic agents are derived from natural products of the *Streptomyces* species of soil fungus. Epirubicin and mitomycin are two examples of such agents, which act at multiple phases of the cell cycle.

7. **The assessment and management of the surgical patient: Clinical decision-making**

A. Preoperative chemoradiation followed by low anterior resection
B. Wide local excision
C. Combined chemoradiotherapy
D. Radical radiotherapy
E. Endocavitary radiotherapy
F. Preoperative radiotherapy followed by low anterior resection
G. Abdominoperineal resection
H. Subtotal colectomy

For each of the following situations, select the single most appropriate treatment from the options listed. Each option may be used once, more than once, or not at all.

1. A 55-year-old male presents to the surgical outpatient clinic with a 2-month history of bleeding per rectum. On examination, a hard, ulcerated growth is palpable over the left lateral wall of the anal canal. The anal sphincter is competent. Biopsy reveals a squamous cell carcinoma of the anal canal. There are no enlarged lymph nodes and no evidence of distant metastasis. What would be the most appropriate management of this patient?

2. A 63-year-old male presents to the surgical outpatient clinic with a 4-month history of bleeding per rectum. Digital rectal examination reveals a 4 x 4 cm hard, proliferative growth in the anal canal approximately 4 cm from the anal verge. The competence of the anal sphincter is lost. Biopsy reveals squamous cell carcinoma. There are no palpable nodes and no evidence of distant metastasis. What would be the most appropriate management of this patient?

3. A 69-year-old male presents to the surgical outpatient clinic with a 6-week history of intermittent rectal bleeding, loss of weight, loss of appetite, and intermittent constipation and diarrhoea. Digital rectal examination reveals a fixed growth 7 cm from the anal verge. Biopsy is suggestive of moderately differentiated adenocarcinoma. CT scan reveals thickening of the wall of the lower rectum with loss of fat plane with the prostate, and perirectal stranding. There are no palpable nodes and no distant metastasis. What would be the most appropriate management of this patient?

8. Perioperative care: Haemostasis and blood products

A. Anaphylaxis
B. Acute haemolytic transfusion reaction
C. Allergic reaction
D. Bacterial contamination
E. Fluid overload
F. Iron overload
G. Hepatitis C
H. Hypocalcaemia
I. Non-haemolytic febrile transfusion reaction
J. Post-transfusion purpura
K. Transfusion-related acute lung injury (TRALI)

For each of the following situations, select the single most likely diagnosis from the options listed. Each option may be used once, more than once, or not at all.

1. A 29-year-old woman admitted to the gynaecological ward receives an elective blood transfusion for symptomatic anaemia secondary to menorrhagia. Nearly 45 minutes after her transfusion is commenced, her temperature rises to 38.7°C and she is found to be shivering. Her pulse rate is 76/min, blood pressure is 122/84 mmHg, and respiratory rate is 14/min with a normal breathing pattern.

2. A 55-year-old woman admitted to the orthopaedic ward following a total hip replacement is receiving a postoperative blood transfusion for anaemia secondary to intraoperative blood loss. Nearly an hour after commencing the transfusion, she is found to have shortness of breath and stridor. On examination, she appears cyanosed with swelling of her face and tongue. Her temperature is 36.8°C, pulse rate is 98/min, and she has an audible wheeze.

3. A 47-year-old man admitted to the surgical admission unit with class III hypovolaemic shock secondary to a road traffic accident complains of pain in his chest and abdomen soon after starting an emergency blood transfusion. He appears agitated and flushed. His temperature is 41.8°C, pulse rate is 102/min, and BP is 94/74 mmHg.

4. A 78-year-old man with moderate rectal bleeding secondary to suspected bowel cancer is receiving his fourth unit of blood as part of his preoperative optimization. He now complains of progressive difficulty in breathing. His temperature is 37.2°C and pulse rate is 76/min but his oxygen saturation has dropped to 87% on air. On examination, his JVP is raised and bilateral basal crepitations are heard on auscultation of his chest.

5. A 25-year-old man of Afro-Caribbean origin, who has had numerous hospital admissions and blood transfusions for sickle cell disease, presents to his GP with progressive tiredness, painful joints and skin pigmentation. Serum biochemistry reveals deranged liver function tests including elevated ALP and ALT levels. A routine urine dipstick test reveals the presence of glucose.

9. **Professional behaviour and leadership: Clinical reasoning**

   A. Immediate A
   B. Immediate B
   C. Urgent—daytime emergency list
   D. Urgent—out-of-hours emergency theatre including night
   E. Expedited
   F. Elective
   G. Does not need surgery
   H. None of the above

   For each of the following situations, select the single most appropriate level of urgency from the options listed. Each option may be used once, more than once, or not at all.

   1. A 30-year-old motorcyclist is involved in a RTA and requires a laparotomy for suspected intra-abdominal haemorrhage.

   2. A 20-year-old female presents with a 48-hour history of acute appendicitis with generalized peritonism.

   3. A 45-year-old male presents with increasing pain and swelling of his left lower leg following reduction and casting of a tibial fracture.

10. **The assessment and management of the surgical patient: Planning investigations**

    A. Rigid sigmoidoscopy
    B. Flexible sigmoidoscopy
    C. Proctoscopy
    D. Colonoscopy
    E. Mesenteric angiography
    F. CT scan
    G. Magnetic resonance imaging
    H. Barium enema
    I. Barium follow-through

    For each of the following situations, select the single most appropriate investigation from the options listed. Each option may be used once, more than once, or not at all.

    1. A 71-year-old man presents to the surgical outpatient clinic with a 2-month history of vague right-sided lower abdominal pain, fatigue, anorexia and weight loss. He also describes a strong family history of bowel cancer. Recent tests requested by his GP reveal that his serum haemoglobin is 8.6 g/dL and his stools are positive for faecal occult blood. What is the most appropriate investigation indicated at this stage?

    2. A 62-year-old woman with no previous medical history presents to the Emergency Department with colicky lower abdominal pain, abdominal bloating, and flatulence. She says that her symptoms settle after defecation. On examination, her abdomen is soft but tenderness is elicited over her left iliac fossa. Digital rectal examination is normal. What is the most appropriate investigation in this patient?

    3. A 71-year-old man with a history of atrial fibrillation presents to the Emergency Department with severe periumbilical pain, vomiting, and loss of appetite. On examination, his pulse is 92/min and BP 118/72 mmHg. Analysis of his arterial blood gas confirms a mild metabolic acidosis and raised serum lactate. Plain radiography of the abdomen obtained 12 hours later reveals 'thumb-printing' of the transverse colon. Assuming that he does not require immediate surgical intervention, which one investigation is most appropriate in this patient?

11. Perioperative care: Preoperative assessment and management

A. ECG only

B. Chest radiography only

C. Renal function, full blood count (FBC), and ECG

D. Renal function, FBC, ECG, and chest radiography

E. FBC and renal function only

F. FBC, renal function, ECG, chest radiography, ABG, and lung function tests

G. No investigations required

H. FBC only

I. Renal function only

For each of the following situations, select the single most appropriate preoperative workup required from the options listed. Each option may be used once, more than once, or not at all.

1. A 30-year-old male with ASA grade 1 is listed for a minor surgical procedure under general anaesthetic. What compulsory preoperative investigations are required for this patient?

2. A 48-year-old man with ASA grade 2 secondary to renal disease is scheduled for a carotid endarterectomy procedure. What compulsory preoperative investigations are required for this patient?

3. An 80-year-old man with ASA grade 2 secondary to cardiovascular disease is scheduled for an anterior resection procedure. What compulsory preoperative investigations are required for this patient?

12. Professional behaviour and leadership: Evidence and guidelines

A. Ia

B. Ib

C. IIa

D. IIb

E. III

F. IV

G. Phase 1 study

H. Phase 2 study

I. Phase 3 study

For each of the following studies, select the single most accurate level of evidence, or trial phase, from the options listed. Each option may be used once, more than once, or not at all.

1. A study was designed to assess the efficacy of neostigmine in the treatment of acute colonic pseudo-obstruction. Patients diagnosed with pseudo-obstruction with a colonic diameter of greater than 10 cm not responding to conservative management were randomized to either 2 mg of neostigmine or saline. The response to the treatment was assessed by a clinician blinded to the treatment given.

2. A medical student published a series of case reports on the association of nicorandil with spontaneous caecal perforation, and wished to know the level of evidence provided by her study.

3. A multicentre cohort study was performed to assess the risks associated with preoperative anaemia in cardiac surgery. All patients who underwent cardiac surgery over a defined period were identified. The prevalence of preoperative anaemia and its adjusted and unadjusted relationships with in-hospital death, acute stroke, and acute kidney injury were identified.

13. **The assessment and management of the surgical patient: Clinical decision-making**

A. Abdominoperineal resection
B. Caecostomy
C. Double-barrel colostomy
D. End colostomy
E. Left hemicolectomy
F. Loop ileostomy
G. Palliative therapy
H. Right hemicolectomy
I. Transverse loop colostomy
J. Total colectomy with end ileostomy

For each of the following situations, select the single most appropriate operative outcome from the options listed. Each option may be used once, more than once, or not at all.

1. An 80-year-old man presents with signs and symptoms of large bowel obstruction. He suffers from ischaemic heart disease and COPD, requiring long-term home oxygen therapy. A CT scan of his abdomen reveals an obstructing left-sided colonic mass that is highly suggestive of a tumour, with likely hepatic and pulmonary metastases.

2. A 57-year-old female presents to the Emergency Department with a 2-day history of progressively worsening left iliac fossa pain, anorexia and swinging pyrexia. An abdominopelvic CT scan confirms the presence of a left pericolic abscess and diverticular mass. She soon becomes peritonitic and undergoes an emergency laparotomy. Intraoperatively, a large amount of pus is found within the pelvis, and is deemed to have originated from perforation of the pericolic abscess.

3. A 49-year-old female presents to the Emergency Department with an acute exacerbation of colitis, which she has been suffering from for over twenty years. She is found to be anaemic and has recently lost a significant amount of weight. Despite a week of inpatient treatment, she continues to experience bloody diarrhoea and is not responding to aggressive medical therapy. A CT scan of her abdomen excludes any intra-abdominal abscesses or toxic megacolon but confirms the presence of extensive colitis.

14. Perioperative care: Preoperative assessment and management

A. Hereditary spherocytosis
B. Iron-deficiency anaemia
C. Thalassaemia
D. Sickle cell trait
E. Anaemia of chronic disease
F. Alcoholism
G. B12 deficiency
H. Aplastic anaemia
I. Sideroblastic anaemia

For each of the following situations, select the single most likely diagnosis from the options listed. Each option may be used once, more than once, or not at all.

1. A 30-year-old Caucasian male is scheduled for an elective laparoscopic cholecystectomy. He attends the preoperative assessment clinic, where it is found that his Hb is 10.5 g/dL, mean corpuscular volume (MCV) 85 fL, and bilirubin is 50 mg/dL. What is the most likely cause of his anaemia?

2. A 38-year-old woman is scheduled for an elective paraumbilical hernia repair. She has no significant past medical history apart from rheumatoid arthritis. Her blood tests at the preoperative assessment clinic reveal a Hb of 10.0 g/dL and MCV of 73 fL. What is the most likely cause of her anaemia?

3. A 40-year-old male with known Crohn's disease is due to have an elective laparoscopic cholecystectomy. Blood tests from the preoperative assessment clinic reveal a Hb of 9.8 g/dL and MCV of 105 fL. What is the most likely cause of his anaemia?

15. The assessment and management of the surgical patient: Differential diagnosis

A. Aortic dissection
B. Diaphragmatic rupture
C. Duodenal rupture
D. Large bowel laceration
E. Liver laceration
F. Pancreatic disruption
G. Small bowel laceration
H. Splenic rupture
I. Tear of superior mesenteric artery

For each of the following situations, select the single most likely diagnosis from the options listed. Each option may be used once, more than once, or not at all.

1. A victim of a road traffic collision is brought into the Emergency Department having sustained injuries to his left thorax and abdomen. Initial assessment reveals that his pulse rate is 130 bpm and BP is 85/60 mmHg. Aggressive fluid resuscitation improves his BP only transiently. Abdominal examination reveals bruising over his left flank, diffuse tenderness with minimal peritoneal signs, and quiet bowel sounds. A chest radiograph shows fracture of two left lower ribs with no associated haemothorax or pneumothorax.

2. A 22-year-old cyclist suffers a head-on collision with a car, throwing her against the handlebars of her cycle. On arrival to the Emergency Department, she complains of severe back pain. She is normotensive but is found to have bilateral flank bruising and upper abdominal tenderness. Plain radiographs exclude free air in the peritoneum and retroperitoneum, and any spinal fractures.

3. A pedestrian is hit by a car travelling at 40 miles/hour. He sustains injuries to his anterior chest and abdomen. On arrival to the Emergency Department, he is tachypnoeic with a respiratory rate of 32 breaths/min. A nasogastric tube is passed as he starts to vomit gastric contents. A chest radiograph is performed and shows a small haemothorax, raised left hemidiaphragm, and the NG tube lying within the left side of the chest.

16. Perioperative care: Critical care

A. 20 mL/kg/day of water, 0.5–0.75 mmol/kg/day of sodium, 0.3–0.5 mmol/kg/day of potassium

B. 0.5 mL/kg/day of water, 2 mmol/kg/day of sodium, 1 mmol/kg/day of potassium

C. 40 mL/kg/day of water, 1–1.5 mmol/kg/day of sodium, 0.6–1 mmol/kg/day of potassium

D. 100 mL/kg/day of water, 3 mmol/kg/day of sodium, 2 mmol/kg/day of potassium

E. 1000 mL + 50 mL/kg of water (per kg over 10 kg), 4 mmol/kg/day of sodium, 2 mmol/kg/day of potassium

F. 1500 mL + 20 mL/kg of water (per kg over 20 kg), 3–5 mmol/kg/day of sodium, 2–4 mmol/kg/day of potassium

G. 2500 mL/day of water, 6 mmol/kg/day of sodium, 4 mmol/kg/day of potassium

H. No intravenous fluids indicated

For each of the following situations, select the single most appropriate form of fluid therapy from the options listed. Each option may be used once, more than once, or not at all.

1. A 50-year-old psychiatric patient is admitted following the ingestion of a coin. She complains of complete dysphagia to saliva but she is not vomiting.

2. A child weighing 3 kg is admitted for a major elective surgical procedure. The surgical house officer is subsequently asked to prescribe maintenance fluids appropriately.

3. A 65-year-old gentleman is on the 'enhanced recovery programme' 3 days after a left hemicolectomy. He is found to be euvolaemic and haemodynamically stable.

17. The assessment and management of the surgical patient: Differential diagnosis

A. Abdominal migraine
B. Acute appendicitis
C. Crohn's disease
D. Diverticulitis
E. Mesenteric adenitis
F. Mittelschmerz
G. Porphyria
H. Somatization disorder
I. Tropical sprue
J. Ulcerative colitis

For each of the following situations, select the single most likely diagnosis from the options listed. Each option may be used once, more than once, or not at all.

1. A 77-year-old man with known diverticular disease presents to the Emergency Department with a 4-hour history of central, colicky abdominal pain, anorexia and nausea. He has not opened his bowels to stool in the last 24 hours. Examination reveals a temperature of 38.5°C and generalized abdominal tenderness, which is worst in the right iliac fossa. His ABGs, FBC, and renal function are within normal limits.

2. A 12-year-old schoolgirl presents to her GP with a 6-month history of non-specific abdominal pain and bloating, associated with headaches, joint pains and back pain. Her BMI is 23, and examination of her abdomen is unremarkable. She mentions that she has been living with her father since her mother died of pancreatic cancer the previous year.

3. A 16-year-old hairdresser presents to her GP with a 3-month history of recurrent abdominal pain. The pain is present before she goes to work, and is associated with vomiting and lethargy. She does not recall experiencing it on weekends and during holidays. Physical examination is largely unremarkable.

18. **Assessment and management of patients with trauma (including the multiply injured patient): Resuscitation and early management**

    A. Defunctioning stoma
    B. Distal pancreatectomy
    C. Drainage of lesser sac using stump or closed suction drains
    D. Laparotomy and packing
    E. Non-surgical management with close observation
    F. Pancreaticoduodenal resection
    G. Primary repair of bleeding artery
    H. Resection and primary anastomosis
    I. Splenectomy

    For each of the following situations, select the single most appropriate operative intervention from the options listed. Each option may be used once, more than once, or not at all.

    1. A 25-year-old man presents to the Emergency Department after falling off a horse and being kicked by the animal in his left flank. On examination, he is haemodynamically stable and diffusely bruised in the left flank, with no signs of peritonism. An abdominal CT scan reveals the presence of a perisplenic haematoma.

    2. A 30-year-old female presents to the Emergency Department after being involved in a road traffic accident, during which she is struck by the vehicle's steering wheel on her upper abdomen. Examination reveals slight haemodynamic instability and generalised abdominal peritonism, leading to an emergency laparotomy. Although significant parenchymal injury is noted, no major pancreatic duct disruption is evident during on-table cholangiography.

    3. A 42-year-old female presents to the Emergency Department after being involved in a road traffic accident. Her examination findings necessitate an emergency laparotomy, during which a mesenteric tear is found, together with dusky discolouration and multiple shear injuries to the small bowel.

19. The assessment and management of the surgical patient: Appropriate prescribing

A. Atracurium
B. Iloprost
C. Metoclopramide
D. Octreotide
E. Omeprazole
F. Oxytocin
G. Papaverine
H. Phenoxybenzamine
I. Prochlorperazine
J. Ranitidine

For each of the following situations, select the single most appropriate drug therapy from the options listed. Each option may be used once, more than once, or not at all.

1. A 26-year-old policewoman is brought to the Emergency Department after being stabbed in the back with a knife. She remains systemically well during history and examination, which do not reveal any abnormal symptoms or signs, apart from the knife wound. A CT scan of abdomen reveals some peripancreatic fluid but is otherwise unremarkable. A joint decision is then made to treat the patient conservatively.

2. A 68-year-old gentleman with a history of poorly-controlled peripheral vascular disease gradually develops critical ischaemia of his right leg. The vascular surgeon on call decides that a femoropopliteal bypass would be the best course of action, considering previously unsuccessful attempts at angioplasty. Intraoperatively, a reverse long saphenous vein graft is used as a conduit but at the end of the procedure, the surgeon is concerned that the graft may not be functioning properly.

3. A 38-year-old schoolteacher presents to her GP with a 3-month history of intermittent headaches, palpitations, flushing and anxiety. Although physical examination reveals no abnormal signs, 24-hour urine collection reveals raised free catecholamines, and a subsequent abdominal CT scan reveals a lesion in the left adrenal gland. The patient is counselled for an urgent laparoscopic adrenalectomy.

20. Basic and applied sciences: Microbiology

A. *Pseudomonas aeruginosa*
B. *Neisseria meningitidis*
C. *Salmonella typhi*
D. *Staphylococcus aureus*
E. *Mycobacterium tuberculosis*
F. *Gonococcus* spp.
G. *Helicobacter pylori*
H. *Haemophilus influenzae*
I. *Streptococcus pneumoniae*

For each of the following situations, select the single most likely causative organism from the options listed. Each option may be used once, more than once, or not at all.

1. A 14-year-old boy undergoes an emergency splenectomy following a road traffic accident. Two days postoperatively, routine observations reveal evidence of a systemic inflammatory response syndrome. Which of the listed organisms are known to cause overwhelming sepsis in such situations?

2. A 68-year-old man with a history of recurrent gastric ulcers presents with a 3-month history of anorexia and weight loss. An upper gastrointestinal endoscopy reveals an ulcerated lesion at the pylorus, which is subsequently confirmed to be gastric adenocarcinoma. Which of the listed organisms is linked with the development of gastric cancer?

3. A 60-year-old diabetic man presents with a 4-week history of intermittent pyrexia and progressively worsening lower back pain. Plain radiography of the lumbar spine confirms the presence of sclerotic bony changes and a marked periosteal reaction. Which of the listed organism is the most likely causative agent?

21. **The assessment and management of the surgical patient: Differential diagnosis**

A. Ulcerative colitis
B. Crohn's disease
C. Angiodysplasia
D. Haemorrhoids
E. Colorectal cancer
F. Pseudomembranous colitis
G. Ischaemic colitis
H. Fissure-in-ano
I. Diverticulosis/diverticulitis

For each of the following situations, select the single most likely diagnosis from the options listed. Each option may be used once, more than once, or not at all.

1. A 28-year-old woman presents to her GP with a 2-month history of progressively worsening perianal pain. She also describes intermittent episodes of diarrhoea with vague abdominal pain. Abdominal examination is unremarkable but rectal examination revealed a chronic fissure at the 12-o'clock position, with a sentinel pile. What is the likely cause of her symptoms?

2. A 40-year-old man presents to the Emergency Department with sudden-onset bloody diarrhoea associated with severe left-sided abdominal pain. He is known to have ankylosing spondylitis but is otherwise fit and well. Examination reveals mild pyrexia with otherwise normal vital signs, and mild left iliac fossa tenderness with no signs of peritonism. What is the likely cause of his symptoms?

3. A 55-year-old gentleman presents to his GP with a 5-day history of worsening left iliac fossa pain. He has experienced intermittent left iliac fossa pain over the last year, associated with constipation, and is currently being treated with repeated courses of antibiotics for recurrent urinary tract infections. Examination reveals normal vital signs and tenderness with guarding in the left iliac fossa and suprapubic region. What is the likely cause of his symptoms?

22. Basic surgical skills: Incisions

A. Gridiron
B. Kocher's
C. Lanz
D. McBurney's
E. Midline laparotomy
F. Paramedian
G. Pfannenstiel
H. Rooftop
I. Rutherford Morrison
J. Thoracoabdominal
K. Transverse

For each of the following situations, select the single most appropriate surgical incision from the options listed. Each option may be used once, more than once, or not at all.

1. A consultant surgeon wishes to perform an elective right hemicolectomy using a particular surgical incision. He tells his medical student that the incision has the advantage of better cosmesis and decreased postoperative pain, albeit at a slightly higher risk of incisional hernia formation.

2. A 45-year-old man presents with back pain and collapse. On examination, he is haemodynamically unstable with an expansile, pulsatile mass in his abdomen. The surgical registrar on call wishes to operate on him immediately.

3. A 16-year-old girl presents with acute appendicitis. The surgeon pays particular attention to minimizing the degree of scarring anticipated from the procedure.

23. The assessment and management of the surgical patient: Appropriate prescribing

A. Paracetamol
B. Codeine
C. Non-steroidal anti-inflammatory drugs and steroids
D. Morphine
E. Cannabis
F. Radiotherapy
G. Chemotherapy
H. Hormone therapy
I. Anticonvulsants and antidepressants

For each of the following situations, select the single most appropriate form of analgesia from the options listed. Each option may be used once, more than once, or not at all.

1. A 78-year-old patient with a recent diagnosis of colon cancer presents to the Emergency Department with severe lower back pain. Plain radiography of the lumbar spine reveals lucent osteolytic lesions within the L3 and L4 vertebral bodies.

2. A 60-year-old female who has previously undergone a right hemicolectomy for colonic malignancy presents to the Emergency Department with right upper quadrant abdominal pain. Her LFTs are found to be deranged and a CT scan of the abdomen reveals the presence of hepatic lesions suggestive of delayed metastasis.

3. A 75-year-old female presents to her GP with shooting pains down her right arm into her fingertips. She has previously undergone curative surgery for breast cancer, although she cannot recall the details of the operation. Examination reveals a hard, fixed mass in the region of her previous tumour, associated with axillary lymphadenopathy.

24. Basic surgical skills: Surgical technique

A. Omental patch
B. Excision of ulcer and closure
C. Billroth I partial gastrectomy
D. Billroth II partial gastrectomy
E. Oversew, omental patch and vagotomy
F. Pylorus-preserving pancreaticoduodenectomy
G. Total gastrectomy with Roux-en-Y reconstruction
H. Oversew, omental patch and pyloroplasty
I. Oversewing of ulcer

For each of the following situations, select the single most appropriate surgical intervention from the options listed. Each option may be used once, more than once, or not at all.

1. An 85-year-old woman undergoes an emergency laparotomy for generalised peritonitis. Intraoperatively, the surgeon notes a 1 cm perforation from an anterior gastric antral ulcer, with sharp, well-defined edges. In addition, significant intra-abdominal contamination is evident.

2. A 30-year-old man undergoes an emergency laparotomy for generalised peritonitis. Intraoperatively, the surgeon notes a 5 mm perforation in the anterior aspect of the duodenum.

3. A 60-year-old man undergoes an emergency laparotomy for generalised peritonitis. Intraoperatively, the surgeon notes a perforated, malignant-looking ulcer in the body of the stomach.

1. Answers: 1-C; 2-E; 3-A

1. Ulcerative colitis is an inflammatory disease of the bowel that usually starts in the rectum and spreads proximally. It is associated with multiple small ulcers in the rectum, which tend to occasionally bleed, thus giving rise to a bloody discharge per rectum. Inflammation of the rectum (proctitis) or colon (colitis) can also lead to an increase in gut mucus production, giving rise to mucus in the stool. The condition is associated with anaemia and hypoproteinaemia. Severe disease is often suggested by: opening of bowels more than four times/day, fever >37.5°C, tachycardia >90/min, hypoalbuminaemia (< 30 g/L), and unintentional weight loss >3 kg. In severe cases, the patient may open their bowels up to 15–20 times/day.

2. Fulminating colitis is a life-threatening complication of inflammatory or infectious colitis. Patients may present with severe abdominal pain and signs of a systemic inflammatory response syndrome (including shock), and even multiple organ dysfunction. This is caused by inflammation of all the muscle layers of the colon. Plain radiography demonstrating a segmental, non-obstructive dilatation of the colon to greater than 6 cm diameter is very suggestive of fulminating colitis. The principles of managing this condition include supportive care in an intensive care environment, keeping the patient 'nil by mouth' (with total parenteral feeding if required), gastric decompression with a nasogastric tube, stoppage of antimotility agents, serial abdominal radiographs and careful monitoring of serum components. General supportive treatment should be administered with intravenous fluids and corticosteroids, while infectious causes of colitis should be treated appropriately. Surgery should be considered for progressive colonic dilatation or worsening systemic toxicity, haemorrhage or perforation.

3. Ischaemic colitis is typically a chronic, segmental process of colonic under-perfusion affecting the watershed areas of the splenic flexure or the rectosigmoid region. It involves transient critical ischaemia of the gut, such as from thromboembolic disease of the superior or inferior mesenteric arteries. The signs and symptoms include a sudden onset of abdominal pain (which is characteristically out of proportion to the clinical signs), vomiting, passage of blood per rectum, and shock. The condition is typically seen in elderly patients with atrial fibrillation, or those with significant systemic atherosclerotic disease. During surgery (i.e. if spontaneous resolution does not occur), areas of haemorrhagic infarction may be noted in the affected segments of colon.

2. Answers: 1-G; 2-B; 3-I

1. Morton's neuroma (or "Morton's metatarsalgia") is a condition associated with a painful but benign neuroma at the level of the metatarsal necks. The common digital nerve to the 3rd/4th metatarsal spaces is most often affected, although other interspaces can be involved. The neuroma is characterized by perineural fibrosis and nerve degeneration due to repetitive irritation, trauma, ischaemia or nerve entrapment. It is seen most frequently in women (female:male = 8:1) aged 40–50, who wear high-heeled, pointed-toe shoes.

The clinical features of Morton's neuroma involve sharp intermittent pain that shoots into the toes, which is usually felt when the patient wears shoes. There is localized tenderness over the site of the neuroma, and diminished sensation in the affected cleft. The patient will often admit to relieving the pain by removing the shoe and manipulating the foot. Radiography is not useful, except to rule out other causes. Treatment involves changing footwear, using arch supports or pads to relieve pressure from the area, and resting the feet. Some patients may require anti-inflammatory drugs, corticosteroid injections, or surgery. Although surgical excision of the neuroma alleviates the pain, it may result in permanent numbness of the affected toes.

2. Bursae are fluid-filled spaces lined by endothelium. They function to permit free movement between opposing tendon, bone, and skin. Bursitis refers to the inflammation of such bursae, which may result from injury, infection, or rheumatoid synovitis. When inflamed, pressure on the joint or movement causes pain. In this case, the patient's signs and symptoms suggest bursitis at the interphalangeal joint of the big toe.

Treatment is usually conservative and includes rest and immobilizing the affected joint. Additionally, the patient may apply ice to reduce the swelling, and take NSAIDs to reduce pain and inflammation. The bursitis usually resolves within 2 weeks, although recurrent flare-ups are common.

3. Tarsal tunnel syndrome may refer to either 'anterior' or 'posterior' tarsal tunnel syndrome.

Anterior tarsal syndrome is a rare entrapment neuropathy involving the terminal portion of the deep peroneal nerve as it runs below the dense superficial fascia of the ankle, resulting in numbness and paraesthesia in the 1st dorsal web space.

Posterior tarsal tunnel syndrome (i.e. in this case) is also uncommon, and results from entrapment of the posterior tibial nerve at the level of the medial malleolus, resulting in pain in the sole. Causative factors include repetitive strain, flat feet, obesity, and any lesion that causes compression of the tibial nerve within the tarsal tunnel region. The diagnosis is usually made clinically by palpating along the course of the nerve in the tarsal tunnel to elicit discomfort either locally or distally, which may be exacerbated by passive pronation of the foot. (Note: the tarsal tunnel is on the medial aspect of the ankle passing from just behind the medial malleolus towards the distal aspect of the calcaneo-navicular region.) In addition, percussion of the nerve may cause symptoms distally (Tinel's sign) or proximally (Valleix phenomenon). Radiography, ultrasonography, and MRI scans may assist in identifying the causative pathology. Despite the widespread use of nerve conduction studies to aid diagnosis, results may often be normal despite the clinical symptoms.

Conservative management (e.g. simple analgesia or analgesia for neurogenic pain; supportive footwear and orthoses; local anaesthetic or corticosteroid injections under nerve stimulator guidance; or radiofrequency lesioning) should be attempted first. Surgical intervention would involve excision of any space-occupying lesions, or tarsal tunnel release.

3. Answers: 1-A; 2-C; 3-G

1. Injuries to the common peroneal nerve (L4–S2) frequently occur following fractures of the neck of the fibula, as in this case. The common peroneal nerve supplies the extensor and peroneal groups of muscles within the leg. The sensory branches supply the anterior and lateral aspect of the leg, and the whole of the dorsum of the foot and toes, except the skin between the great and the 2nd toe—this is supplied by the deep peroneal nerve. Injury to this nerve results in foot drop and sensory loss over the anterior and lateral aspect of the leg, the dorsum of the foot and the toes.

2. The lateral cutaneous nerve of the thigh passes from the lateral border of psoas major across the iliac fossa to pierce the inguinal ligament. It travels in a fibrous tunnel medial to the anterior superior iliac spine and enters the thigh deep to the fascia lata before continuing distally into the

subcutaneous tissues. The nerve can have one of three origins (i.e. L1/L2, L2/L3, or L3 alone); it divides into its anterior and posterior branches just distal to the inguinal ligament and supplies the anterolateral aspect of the thigh. Compression of the nerve as it passes through the inguinal ligament (or as it pierces the fascia lata) causes meralgia paraesthetica (or Roth's meralgia). Although this is common following many orthopaedic procedures, non-surgical causes include seat belts, tight trousers, obesity, pregnancy, intra-abdominal or intrapelvic pathology, diabetes mellitus, alcoholism, lead poisoning, or spontaneous occurrence. Patients characteristically describe a burning or stinging sensation over the anterolateral aspect of the thigh, which is aggravated by walking or standing, and is relieved by lying down with the hip flexed. These symptoms are usually self-limiting but local nerve blocks may be beneficial. Surgical intervention should be restricted to freeing the nerve, as division may aggravate the original symptoms.

3. The sciatic nerve (L4–S2) supplies the hamstrings and all the muscles of the leg and foot via the tibial and common peroneal nerves. It also supplies sensation to the lateral part of the leg below the knee, including the foot. Injury to the sciatic nerve is common following total hip replacement, posterior dislocation of the hip, or any other form of hip trauma. Other causes include misplaced gluteal injections, pelvic disease, and, very rarely, nerve entrapment. The clinical manifestations of sciatic nerve palsy reflect its motor and sensory distribution and may include foot drop; loss of power below the knee and loss of knee flexion; loss of ankle jerk and plantar reflexes (but not knee jerk); and loss of sensation below the knee on the lateral side of the leg. Treatment involves wearing shoes with plastic inserts during the day, and aluminium 'night shoes' at night, to prevent foot drop and contracture of the calf musculature.

4. Answers: 1-G; 2-D; 3-E

1. Early postoperative obstruction is rare, but when it does occur, it presents with colicky abdominal pain, distension, vomiting, and absolute constipation. Bowel sounds are usually hyperactive and high-pitched. It may be caused by a loop of bowel becoming twisted or trapped within a peritoneal defect or omental window which is inadvertently (or inevitably) created during laparotomy or laparoscopy. It may also be the result of a missed band adhesion. Fibrinous adhesions may also cause obstruction—this usually develops one week after an operation. Both cases may be transient and settle with nasogastric tube drainage and intravenous fluid rehydration. A small proportion of patients will develop fulminant intestinal obstruction with tenderness and systemic signs of toxicity, which warrants a reoperation. It should be noted that postoperative ileus may also result from prolonged surgical manipulation of the small bowel.

2. Anastomotic leakage usually occurs between postoperative days 3 and 7. It is one of the most important complications of bowel surgery as delayed diagnosis and intervention may lead to sepsis, multiorgan dysfunction, and fistula formation. Small leaks are relatively common—they commonly progress to form localized abscesses and can be treated conservatively. Major anastomotic leaks can cause peritonitis and large intra-abdominal abscesses, which present with swinging pyrexia and other features of systemic sepsis. These patients usually need reoperation with drainage of the abscess, and the two ends of the anastomosis brought out as temporary stomas.

3. A fistula is an abnormal connection between two epithelial surfaces. Enterocutaneous fistulas most commonly develop as a complication of bowel surgery. In the postoperative setting, the causes of fistulas include anastomotic leak, bowel ischaemia, unintentional enterotomy, or inadvertent small bowel injury at the time of closure. In this scenario, the presence of gas and offensive feculent discharge from the wound is an indication of an underlying fistula. The cause may be a 'blown appendix stump', inadvertent enterotomy, or even an underlying inflammatory pathology such as Crohn's disease, particularly with a history of recurrent right iliac fossa pain and a macroscopically normal-looking appendix.

5. Answers: 1-J; 2-F; 3-A

1. Tracheobronchial injury is a rare but potentially fatal consequence of either blunt or penetrating trauma to the neck and chest. It may present in a similar fashion as described scenario. An endotracheal tube should be inserted to ensure the airway remains patent. Definitive diagnosis requires bronchoscopy to visualize the airway, and thorough radiographic workup. Almost all patients with traumatic tracheobronchial injuries require surgical repair and should therefore be referred for urgent cardiothoracic assessment.

2. Oesophageal perforations are uncommon and usually occur after instrumentation. The perforations that occur following external trauma are more likely to be due to penetrating injury rather than blunt injury. Traumatic ruptures are more likely to happen in the cervical oesophagus and result in leakage of saliva, food, and bile, resulting in mediastinitis (and potential necrosis), severe sepsis and death in up to 30% of cases. Persistent vomiting, chest pain and subcutaneous emphysema are the triad of clinical findings classically expected in oesophageal perforation. Management within the Emergency Department should include oxygen, intravenous antibiotics, intravenous fluids, opioid analgesia, nasogastric tube placement and surgical chest drains to remove gastric contents and pus from the chest. Small well-defined tears can be treated conservatively, whereas larger tears should undergo urgent repair in patients who are fit for surgery.

3. Traumatic aortic dissection is often the result of deceleration injury causing rotatory avulsion of the aortic arch. Dissection of the descending aorta presents with tearing back pain while anterior chest pain is the predominant symptom of a dissecting ascending aorta. Clinical findings include asymmetry in brachial artery pressures (i.e. a difference of systolic blood pressure of > 20 mmHg between both arms) and peripheral hypoperfusion. Radiographic findings of a widened mediastinum, small pleural effusion and deviated trachea are highly suggestive, and should be followed by a CT scan of the thorax to confirm the presence and extent of aortic dissection. Management depends largely on the originating site and extent of dissection within the aorta. Surgery is indicated in all patients with type A dissection (i.e. dissection of the ascending aorta with or without extension to the descending aorta)—without surgery, the 48-hour mortality is as high as 50%. Surgery involves a Dacron tube graft being inserted, via an open or endovascular approach, to replace the affected length of the aorta, and occasionally extending beyond the arch. In contrast, the ideal management of type B dissection (i.e. dissection that is confined to the descending aorta) is less clear, and surgery is indicated only when complications develop after the institution of medical therapy. The aims of drug therapy include maintaining a reduction in systemic blood pressure (e.g. with beta-blockers and nitro-vasodilators). In addition, patients should have their clinical parameters closely monitored in an intensive care setting until initial recovery is evident.

6. Answers: 1-A; 2-C; 3-B

1. As malignant cells proliferate at increased rates, they spend less time in the error-correction phase and are therefore at a higher risk of death from DNA damage. Alkylating agents are similarly toxic to normal cells, causing damage particularly to high-turnover cells such as those of the gastrointestinal tract, bone marrow and genitals. These agents can be classified into mustard gas derivatives (melphalan, cyclophosphamide), ethylenimines, alkylsulphonates (busulphan), hydrazines, nitrosurease, and metal salts (cisplatin, carboplatin).

2. Purine and pyrimidine analogues become integrated into a cell's DNA configuration as a substitute for its genuine constituents during the S phase, halting normal cell division. In a similar way, antimetabolites are classified according to the substances with which they interfere at specific phases of the cell cycle. These include:

- Folic acid antagonists: methotrexate
- Pyrimidine analogues: 5-fluorouracil, capecitabine

- Purine analogues: 6-mercaptopurine
- Adenosine deaminase inhibitors: cladribine

3. Anti-tumour antibiotics are chemotherapeutic agents derived from natural products of the *Streptomyces* species of soil fungi, with varied mechanisms of action. For example, the actinomycins act by binding to DNA and inhibiting DNA-dependent RNA synthesis, while the anthracyclins intercalate between base pairs and inhibit RNA and DNA synthesis. In contrast, the bleomycin peptide acts by reacting with DNA and separating its strands. Nevertheless, it is the collective mode of action of all of the above agents on tumour cell DNA that is responsible for their recognised chemotherapeutic effects.

7. Answers: 1-C; 2-G; 3-A

1. Combined chemoradiation therapy is the first line of management in patients with squamous cell carcinoma of anal canal but with a competent anal sphincter. This combined modality treatment results in higher rates of both local control and survival, and preservation of anal function when compared to surgery.

2. Surgery, in the form of abdominoperineal resection, is the most appropriate form of management for squamous cell carcinoma of the anal canal that has destroyed the competence of the anal sphincter. Eradication of the tumour by chemoradiotherapy does not restore continence since the cancer cells are replaced with fibrous tissue rather than the specialized muscle tissue of the anal sphincters. Another factor making this option preferable to chemoradiotherapy and low anterior resection is the proximity of the tumour to the anal verge (i.e. 6 cm is generally considered to be the cut-off point for selection between abdominoperineal resection and low anterior resection).

3. The two important end-points in preoperative chemoradiotherapy are: (1) evidence of tumour downstaging and (2) long-term disease control. The addition of concurrent chemotherapy along with radiation increases the pathological complete response rate to about 15–30% as opposed to less than 10% with preoperative radiotherapy alone. Randomized studies have suggested better local tumour control for T3/T4 tumours by using preoperative chemoradiotherapy. The proximity of the tumour from the anal verge also suggests that low anterior resection may be considered over abdominoperineal resection (see explanation (2)).

8. Answers: 1-I; 2-A; 3-B; 4-E; 5-F

1. The clinical findings in this patient are suggestive of a non-haemolytic febrile transfusion reaction. This is primarily because the patient has a temperature of less than 40°C with shivers but all other physiological parameters are within normal limits.

2. This patient has an anaphylactic reaction to blood transfusion. Such patients present with oedema of tongue, cyanosis, dyspnoea (from bronchospasm) and tachycardia. Transfusion should be discontinued immediately if the patient develops such signs. The patient should be appropriately resuscitated and treated. This consists of administering high-flow oxygen, securing intravenous access, and administration of an antihistamine (e.g. chlorpheniramine maleate) and a steroid (e.g. hydrocortisone). The use of adrenaline may also be indicated in some patients.

3. This patient has all the signs and symptoms suggestive of an acute haemolytic transfusion reaction (temperature >40°C, chest and/or abdominal pain, tachycardia, hypotension, agitation and flushing). Acute haemolytic transfusion reactions may be caused by ABO incompatibility. In such cases, the transfusion should be stopped immediately, and the patient should be appropriately resuscitated. All remaining blood products should be returned to the laboratory for further analysis.

4. The signs and symptoms in this patient are suggestive of pulmonary oedema secondary to fluid overload. This can occur if the patient is transfused rapidly or receives large volumes of blood in a relatively short period of time. This typically occurs in elderly patients who may have concurrent medical comorbidities, such as a compromised cardiac status, hypertension or renal dysfunction. The features of pulmonary oedema, amongst others, include shortness of breath, a raised JVP, bibasal lung crepitations, and a drop in oxygen saturation.

5. This patient is manifesting the symptoms of iron overload (i.e. secondary haemochromatosis) which has developed as a result of repeated blood transfusions for sickle cell disease. Secondary haemochromatosis may occur in any haematological condition where the patient has received repeated blood transfusions. Features of haemochromatosis include tiredness, arthralgia, diabetes mellitus, deranged LFTs and associated signs of chronic liver disease, bronze skin pigmentation, dilated cardiomyopathy, and hypogonadism.

9. Answers: 1-A; 2-D; 3-B

The NCEPOD (National Confidential Enquiry into Perioperative Deaths) classification was introduced to ensure that patients are operated on within the time frame appropriate for their condition and to ensure that medical staff are operating out-of-hours only when it is appropriate.

1. Immediate A category is usually for life-saving operations, where patients should be resuscitated simultaneously with surgical treatment. The procedure should be undertaken within minutes of the decision being made. This will sometimes require 'breaking into' existing lists, e.g. leaking abdominal aortic aneurysm (AAA), major thoracoabdominal trauma.

2. Urgent—out-of-hours emergency theatre including night is the level of urgency for acute-onset conditions which, if deteriorate, threaten life, limb, or organs. The procedure should take place once resuscitation is complete, within hours of the decision being made.

3. Immediate B: same as (1) but described a limb- or organ-saving intervention and should be performed within minutes.

10. Answers: 1-D; 2-D; 3-E

1. This patient, in view of his age, history, anaemia, and positive faecal occult blood, is likely to have a colonic malignancy. The clinical presentation of patients with colonic malignancy depends on the site of the tumour. Right-sided colonic carcinoma commonly presents with anaemia, tiredness, malaise, pallor, and loss of weight, while left-sided colonic carcinoma may more often present with altered bowel habit, rectal bleeding, tenesmus (mainly from rectal carcinoma), and intestinal obstruction. The most appropriate investigation in this patient would be a colonoscopy since it can visualize the colon up to the caecum.

2. This patient has diverticular disease (i.e. symptomatic diverticulosis), which is characterized by non-specific attacks of abdominal pain, mainly over the left iliac fossa, flatulence, bloating, and alternating constipation and diarrhoea. The pain is colicky in nature and is often relieved by passing flatus or after defecation. In patients with a history suggestive of diverticular disease, barium enema used to be the first-line investigation but has now been superseded by endoscopy in most centres. Although flexible sigmoidoscopy is sufficient to diagnose diverticular disease, this patient's age and the associated risk of colorectal malignancy warrants colonoscopy as the first-line investigation, where resources permit. This may be supplemented by a CT scan of the abdomen. A potentially useful, novel virtual imaging modality is CT colonography but the evidence supporting its utility in diverticular disease is still limited.

3. It is highly likely that this patient has developed acute mesenteric ischaemia, which results from a sudden decrease in intestinal perfusion, and is common in elderly patients who are in atrial

fibrillation. The typical presentation of mesenteric ischaemia is with severe periumbilical or central abdominal pain that is disproportionate to the clinical findings. The accurate clinical diagnosis of this condition is therefore a challenging one to make. In the later stages, plain abdominal radiography may reveal 'thumb-printing' of the gut wall, which is caused by interstitial oedema with haemorrhage in the affected segment. Mesenteric angiography, to identify the emboli or thrombi, localize vascular obstructions, and characterize the collateral circulation, is the investigation of choice to diagnose suspected mesenteric ischaemia in those who do not have signs of perforation or peritonitis.

11. Answers: 1-G; 2-C; 3-D

Although the following explanations include the recommended use of the National Institute for Health and Clinical Excellence (NICE) guidelines in perioperative care, it must be understood that these are simply guidelines and not mandatory protocols. They must be used in conjunction with local institutional policy, as well as expert (i.e. consultant) consensus.

1. Fit and healthy patients (ASA grade 1) between ages 16 and 39 undergoing minor procedures do not usually require any routine preoperative investigation. ECG is mandatory in all above 40 years of age and in any patient with cardiovascular comorbidity.

2. FBC and renal function are mandatory investigations for any patient with comorbidity undergoing grade 2 surgery or higher and in all patients more than 60 years of age. ECG is mandatory in all patients above 40 years of age or cardiovascular comorbidity. Checking of clotting screen should be considered in ASA 2 patients with renal impairment. Chest radiography can be considered as per NICE guidelines but is not mandatory.

3. FBC, renal function, and ECG are recommended for this patient. NICE guidance recommends that the benefit of a chest radiograph in patients above the age of 40, with ASA grade 2 and above secondary to cardiovascular or respiratory disease, undergoing grade 2 and above surgery, depends on specific patient characteristics. In practice, a chest radiograph is warranted for this particular patient, given his ASA grade 2 status secondary to cardiovascular disease. Lung function tests and ABGs can be considered, as per NICE guidelines.

12. Answers: 1-B; 2-E; 3-D

The strength of evidence obtained from clinical trials or other forms of research studies is ranked according to the study design and the endpoints measured:

    Ia Evidence from Meta-analysis of Randomised Controlled Trials
    Ib Evidence from at least one Randomised Controlled Trial
    IIa Evidence from at least one well-designed controlled trial, which is not randomised
    IIb Evidence from at least one well-designed experimental trial
    III Evidence from case, correlation, and comparative studies
    IV Evidence from expert opinion

1. This is an example of a randomized controlled trial (RCT), which provides level Ib evidence. Participants in RCTs are randomly allocated to one form of intervention or another, and this can be conducted on a single-blind or double-blind basis. The effects of the experimental intervention are compared against those of the control intervention, frequently representing the comparison of new treatments against current best practices.

2. Case reports, case series, well-designed non-experimental descriptive studies and correlation studies all offer level III evidence. They often employ a simpler form of study design and may be cheaper to conduct than studies ranked higher in the hierarchy of evidence.

3. This describes a cohort study, which, similar to case-control studies, offers level IIb evidence. The highest form of evidence is level Ia, which may be derived from a meta-analysis of RCTs. Level IIa is provided by non-randomized control studies and level IV is based upon expert committee reviews or the opinions of respected authorities.

13. Answers: 1-G; 2-D; 3-J

1. This patient is currently unfit for surgery and is unlikely to be able to manage a stoma. Palliative therapy (e.g. by stenting) is therefore the most appropriate treatment modality. If the patient was fit for surgery (and potentially tolerant of a stoma), transverse loop colostomy may be performed as a last resort, for high left-sided colonic tumours; this would serve to relieve the obstruction and divert faeces away from it. The procedure may also be employed to defunction a diseased segment of distal colon (e.g. for diverticular abscess or colovesical fistula). If the ileocaecal valve is incompetent, loop ileostomy would be preferred for this purpose.

2. A Hartman's procedure involves the diseased segment of rectosigmoid bowel being resected and the proximal end being brought out as an end colostomy, with the distal end closed off and left in situ (i.e. as a rectal stump). This is usually intended to be reversed at a later date, once the patient has recovered from the initial insult of injury and subsequent surgery. It is unfavourable to perform a primary anastomosis in this lady due to the degree of peritoneal contamination encountered, which significantly increases the risk of infection and subsequent anastomotic leakage.

3. Extensive ulcerative colitis that is unresponsive to medical management should be considered for surgical intervention, which is required in 20% of patients with ulcerative colitis. Postoperatively, a significant improvement in quality of life can be expected; a colectomy eliminates the need for continuous medical therapy and the need for cancer surveillance. In addition, most extraintestinal manifestations of ulcerative colitis will resolve after a colectomy—the exceptions to this are sclerosing cholangitis and the enteropathic spondyloarthropathies. Although the acute setting traditionally favoured procedures such as panproctocolectomy and ileostomy formation, it must be noted that restorative proctocolectomy with ileal pouch-anal anastomosis conserves the anal route of defaecation (i.e. without needing a stoma), has become the recent gold standard for surgery in patients with ulcerative colitis.

14. Answers: 1-A; 2-E; 3-G

Anaemia is caused by reduced numbers of red blood cells (RBCs) and/or low Hb concentration, relative to levels that are expected for a person's age and sex.

Anaemia can be due to reduced production or increased destruction/loss of haemoglobin or RBCs.

The most common cause of anaemia worldwide is iron deficiency. This may be caused by blood loss (e.g. menstruation), increased demand for iron (e.g. pregnancy), or poor diet or gastrointestinal (GI) absorption.

Other causes of reduced RBC production include vitamin B12, folate deficiency and bone marrow failure.

Increased destruction of RBCs is largely due to haemolysis. It is classified as congenital (e.g. hereditary spherocytosis, thalassaemia) or acquired. Acquired causes are either immune-mediated or non-immune (e.g. drugs, mechanical valves, malaria).

Hereditary spherocytosis may lead to anaemia due to haemolysis, which also leads to raised serum bilirubin and increases the risk of pigment gallstone formation.

Chronic illnesses such as rheumatoid arthritis may lead to a normocytic or microcytic anaemia (i.e. 'anaemia of chronic disease'), via various mechanisms including bone marrow suppression.

Crohn's disease can affect the terminal ileal absorption of B12, leading to megaloblastic anaemia. The chart shown in Figure 2.1 depicts the classification of anaemia on the basis of mean corpuscular volume.

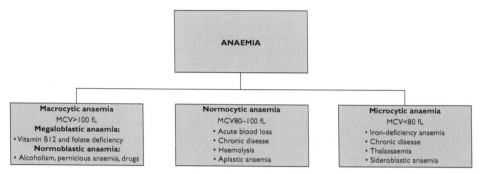

Figure 2.1 Classification of anaemia on the basis of mean corpuscular volume (MCV).

15. Answers: 1-H; 2-F; 3-B

1. Splenic injury usually results from blunt abdominal trauma and is commonly associated with major rib fractures. It may present as per the described scenario, as either a conscious or unconscious patient, with signs of peritonism. However, the main signs are those of haemorrhage. The investigations depend upon whether or not the patient is haemodynamically stable and the management depends upon the degree of injury. If the patient is unstable, laparotomy and possible splenectomy is indicated after initial attempts to resuscitate. Long-term prophylaxis against encapsulated organisms is essential to prevent postsplenectomy sepsis. If the patient is stable, the diagnosis and the extent of injury can be assessed by CT imaging of the abdomen and pelvis. Conservative management is commonly preferred unless there are signs of continuous haemorrhage.

2. Pancreatic disruption usually occurs following compression against the vertebral column from a direct blow or from a deceleration injury. The symptoms are usually masked, the amylase levels are highly variable, and the plain abdominal radiograph may show associated injury to the duodenum as free air within the retroperitoneum. It is most commonly diagnosed during the secondary survey, and on review of the CT scan. Pancreatic disruption may be classified as follows:

- Major injury: proximal gland damage involving head and duct disruption
- Intermediate injury: distal gland damage with duct disruption
- Minor injury: contusion or lacerations which are not associated with any damage to major ducts.

Surgical intervention with pancreaticoduodenectomy is reserved for major proximal injuries.

3. Diaphragmatic rupture usually results from violent abdominal compression following a restrained road traffic collision. On a chest radiograph, a right-sided rupture may appear as a raised right hemidiaphragm, while a left-sided rupture would result in the stomach bubble being visible within the left hemithorax. A more accurate diagnosis can be made on thoracoabdominal CT scanning. Surgical repair is indicated if respiratory function is compromised, or in young patients, to prevent delayed pulmonary complications.

16. Answers: 1-C; 2-D; 3-H

1. This adult patient should be prescribed fluids containing the daily maintenance requirements for water and electrolytes. For the average 70 kg male, this would amount to 2800 mL of water, 105 mmol of sodium, and in the absence of renal disease or hyperkalaemia, 70 mmol of potassium. These maintenance requirements should be tailored to correct deficit or ongoing losses, which the patient in this scenario does have (i.e. she is not vomiting, etc.)

2. Maintenance fluid requirements for the paediatric population can be estimated based on body weight:

- 0–10 kg: 100 mL/kg
- 10–20 kg: 1000 mL + 50 mL/kg for each kg over 10 kg
- >20 kg: 1500 mL + 25 mL/kg for each kg over 20 kg

Electrolyte requirements for maintenance purposes in a healthy child include 2–3 mmol/kg/day of sodium, 1–3 mmol/kg/day of potassium, 2–3 mmol/kg/day of phosphate, 1–2 mmol/kg/day of calcium, and 0.25–0.5 mmol/kg/day of magnesium. For children over the age of 6 months, 10% dextrose with 0.45% normal saline may be used.

3. In patients who are euvolaemic and haemodynamically stable, oral fluid administration should be achieved as soon as possible. Much of the postoperative morbidity associated with fluid replacement is due to the overcompensation of hypovolaemia. Excessive fluid retention leads to tissue oedema and poor wound healing, compromised pulmonary function, bowel oedema and delayed resumption of bowel function. The concept of enhanced recovery therefore recommends intraoperative and postoperative fluid restriction in major colonic surgery with careful avoidance of hypovolaemia.

17. Answers: 1-B; 2-H; 3-A

It is important for surgeons to understand both the surgical and 'non-surgical' causes of abdominal pain. This will facilitate the prompt diagnosis and management of any patient presenting to the Emergency Department with abdominal pain, who the general surgeon on call will likely be requested to review.

1. Despite this gentleman's past medical history of diverticular disease, his signs and symptoms are suggestive of acute appendicitis. The Alvarado score is a widely used tool in estimating the clinical likelihood of acute appendicitis based on symptoms, signs, and initial investigations:

- Migratory right iliac fossa pain (1)
- Nausea or vomiting (1)
- Anorexia (1)
- Right iliac fossa tenderness (2)
- Rebound tenderness (1)
- Elevated temperature >37.3°C (1)
- Leucocytosis (2)
- 'Left shift' of white cells or neutrophilia (1)

Reprinted from Annals of Emergency Medicine, 15, 5, Alfredo Alvarado, 'A practical score for the early diagnosis of acute appendicitis', pp. 557–564. Copyright 1986, with permission from Elsevier.

A total score (from the sum of numbers in brackets) of 5 or 6 is compatible with the diagnosis of acute appendicitis; 7 or 8 indicates probable appendicitis; and 9 or 10 indicates a high probability of acute appendicitis. It is also important to note that the peak incidence of acute appendicitis follows a bimodal distribution (i.e. the young and the elderly). Particularly in the elderly, leucocytosis may not be evident and so a clinical diagnosis of appendicitis often has to be made, although diagnostic laparoscopy is increasingly viewed as an option. Alternatively, abdominal CT scanning can be used to exclude perforation or complications of neoplastic disease, and to confirm the diagnosis.

2. As much as this case seems 'non-surgical' in nature, a reasonable understanding of psychosomatic disease will allow the surgeon to comprehend such ambiguous presentations. Somatization in the young involves persistent somatic distress that may not be compatible with the clinical diagnosis of organic disease. It is often a consequence of psychosocial stress and commonly persists after the acute stressor has resolved. This often leaves children and parents searching for an accurate medical diagnosis, resulting in repeated consultations. In this scenario, the mother's death is a likely precipitating factor. The following criteria are required for the diagnosis of somatization:

- Four different sites of pain (e.g. head, abdomen, back, joints, extremities, chest, rectum) or disturbance of function (e.g. menstruation, sexual intercourse, urination)
- Two gastrointestinal symptoms other than pain (e.g. nausea, bloating or vomiting that is not associated with diarrhoea; intolerance of several different foods)
- One sexual or reproductive symptom other than pain
- One pseudo-neurological symptom (e.g. ataxia, paralysis, aphonia, urinary retention)

3. As in the previous case, this patient's presentation suggests a functional cause for her symptoms. Abdominal migraine, which is a variant of cyclical vomiting syndrome, occurs most frequently in adolescents. Affected patients tend to have violent and occasionally prolonged episodes of vomiting that may be precipitated by stress, concurrent infections or menses. Approximately 80% of patients have prodromal symptoms including nausea, headache, fever, emotional withdrawal, lethargy, sleep pattern changes, and crying. Although the pathophysiology of cyclical vomiting syndrome is unknown, various endogenous factors such as corticotropin-releasing factor and a heightened sympathetic response have been suggested to play a role. A strong genetic component has also been suggested, with evidence of mitochondrial heteroplasmies that predispose to cyclic vomiting syndrome and other related disorders, such as migraine and chronic fatigue syndrome.

18. Answers: 1-E; 2-C; 3-H

1. The spleen is an important immunological and reticuloendothelial organ which should be preserved in children and young adults whenever possible. Following splenic trauma, if the patient is haemodynamically stable with minimal physical abdominal signs, blood transfusion requirements of less than 2 units, or a negative diagnostic peritoneal lavage, he/she should be managed conservatively. Conservative management involves observing for vital parameters, regular abdominal examination, assessing transfusion requirements, and repeating radiological investigations.

2. Pancreatic injuries are rare but when they do occur, they pose difficult management issues due to associated injuries to the surrounding major vessels, extrahepatic biliary system, and the duodenum. The most important aspects of managing pancreatic injuries include the assessment for pancreatic duct and duodenal injuries. During laparotomy, this can be achieved by performing on-table pancreaticography and full mobilization of the duodenum, respectively. Parenchymal damage in the absence of duct injury should be treated by draining the lesser sac using stump or closed suction drains. In haemodynamically stable patients, severe body or tail parenchymal injuries associated with duct injuries warrant a pancreatectomy. Pancreaticoduodenal resection is warranted in patients with proximal duct injury, injuries to the head of the pancreas involving the ampulla, or in situations where the pancreas and the duodenum are devascularized.

3. Major vascular injuries such as mesenteric tears usually present with haemorrhage and hypotension. The management of vascular injuries involves proximal and distal control of the bleeding

vessel to minimize the haemorrhage until the damage can be inspected. In this case the small bowel appears dusky, suggesting ischaemia. This should be managed by resection of the non-viable bowel and primary anastomosis in the absence of contamination.

19. Answers: 1-D; 2-G; 3-H

1. In such cases of isolated, penetrating trauma to the flanks or back, wound exploration is not indicated in the first instance if the patient is stable. It may also prove unreliable and unnecessary due to the strong musculature involved, which makes any tract difficult to predict or to follow. Local wound exploration may also result in further injury or may restart any arrested haemorrhage. Considering that this patient remains stable, CT scanning of the abdomen is indicated to delineate the extent of trauma and quantify potential collateral damage. The peripancreatic fluid collection in this case is almost certainly a result of direct trauma to the pancreas. Conservative treatment is warranted by using octreotide (an analogue of the hypothalamic release-inhibiting hormone, somatostatin), which reduces pancreatic exocrine secretions. It would also be prudent to avoid undue pancreatic stimulation by keeping the patient nil by mouth.

2. Papaverine is an antispasmodic drug that is used primarily in the treatment of visceral spasm (e.g. of the GI tract, bile ducts, ureter), vasospasm (e.g. cerebral, especially in subarachnoid haemorrhage, and arterial bypass surgery), and occasionally, for erectile dysfunction. Its use before or after vein harvesting has been shown to be beneficial, through its mechanism of smooth muscle relaxation, which prevents vigorous, prolonged contracture of the vein. This in turn prevents endothelial sloughing and improved periprocedural vascular patency. This patient will nonetheless require close postoperative observation on the ward to ensure that the graft remains clinically viable.

3. The history and investigative findings in this case are typical of phaeochromocytoma, which is a rare catecholamine-secreting adrenal tumour (usually of the adrenal medulla).These tumours somewhat follow the '10% rule': 10% are malignant, 10% are extra-adrenal, 10% are bilateral, and 10% are familial. Biochemical confirmation of diagnosis may be obtained from measuring 24-hour urinary free catecholamines or vanillylmandelic acid (VMA), or urinary/plasma metanephrines. This should be followed by imaging (CT/MRI) for tumour localization to facilitate preoperative treatment planning. Surgical tumour excision forms the mainstay of treatment but in order to prevent excessive release of catecholamines during the procedure, the patient requires alpha-blockade with phenoxybenzamine, followed by adequate beta-blockade. It is vital that alpha-blockade is established before the introduction of beta-blockade, to prevent inadvertent hypertensive crises (i.e. from unopposed alpha-adrenergic stimulation).

20. Answers: 1-I; 2-G; 3-D

1. Asplenic individuals are at an increased risk of infection from encapsulated organisms such as *Streptococcus pneumoniae*, *Neisseria meningitidis* and *Haemophilus influenzae*. The commonest of these is *Streptococcus pneumoniae*. It is for this reason that all splenectomised patients and those with functional hyposplenism should receive the following prophylactic measures:

- pneumococcal immunisation – ideally, 4-6 weeks before elective splenectomy
- patients not previously immunised should receive *Haemophilus influenzae* type b vaccine
- patients not previously immunised should receive *Meningococcal* group C conjugate vaccine
- annual influenza immunisation
- lifelong amoxicillin (or erythromycin, if allergic to penicillin)

2. *Helicobacter* pylori is a spiral-shaped pathogen that is found in the lining of the stomach in two-thirds of the world's population. It is linked with an increased risk of developing gastric

cancer and gastric mucosa-associated T-cell lymphoma, whilst decreasing the risk of oesophageal cancers in some individuals. The eradication of H. pylori may lead to a moderate reduction in the incidence of gastric cancer.

3. Osteomyelitis is an infection of the bone characterized by pain, localized swelling and pyrexia. The route of infection may either be by direct inoculation or by haematogenous spread. Diabetics and immune-compromised patients are at an increased risk of such infection. Radiological changes occur approximately 10 days after onset, and consist of soft tissue swelling and periosteal elevation. *Staphylococcus aureus* is the most common pathogen in adults, *Haemophilus influenzae* in children, and *Salmonella spp.* in sickle cell patients.

21. Answers: 1-B; 2-A; 3-I

1. Crohn's disease is an idiopathic, chronic, transmural inflammatory bowel disease that can affect any part of the GI tract from mouth to anus. It usually presents with abdominal pain and diarrhoea, which may be bloody in the presence of colitis. It can also present with symptoms of acute or subacute intestinal obstruction due to stricture formation. Crohn's disease and ulcerative colitis may both be associated with extra-intestinal manifestations. Perianal disease (fissures, fistulae, abscesses, and rectal prolapse), eye manifestations (conjunctivitis, iritis, uveitis, and episcleritis), arthritis and gallstones are much more commonly seen in patients with Crohn's disease. Perianal Crohn's disease is seen in 30% of patients and may precede the development of intestinal symptoms.

2. Ulcerative colitis is an idiopathic, acute or chronic inflammatory bowel disease originating in the mucosa and submucosa of the large intestine. It usually presents with abdominal pain, bloody diarrhoea with or without fever, and features of systemic sepsis. Relapsing intermittent procto-colitis typically presents as attacks of increasing frequency and urgency of bloody, loose stools with interspersed normal bowel function. Any attack can progress to fulminant colitis, which is characterized by colonic dilatation, severe systemic upset, increased risk of perforation, and severe haemorrhage. Skin manifestations (e.g. erythema nodosum and pyoderma gangrenosum), ankylosing spondylitis, sacroiliitis, and primary sclerosing cholangitis are more commonly seen in patients with ulcerative colitis.

3. Colonic diverticulae represent outpouchings of the colonic wall containing only mucosa, sub-mucosa, and a serosal covering. They are commonest in the sigmoid and descending colon and almost never occur in the rectum. They can present as painful diverticular disease (i.e. with inter-mittent left iliac fossa pain), rectal bleeding, acute diverticulitis (i.e. gradual-onset left iliac fossa pain with fever and anorexia), complicated acute diverticulitis (i.e. with peri/paracolic abscess formation or peritonitis), large bowel obstruction (i.e. due to an acute inflammatory mass on a background of chronic scarring), chronic diverticulitis, or diverticular fistulae. Diverticular fistulae usually occur with the rupture of a paracolic abscess into adjacent organs; and diverticular fistulae involving the bladder often result in recurrent enteric organism-related urinary tract infections.

22. Answers: 1-K; 2-E; 3-C

1. The transverse incision can be utilized for surgery to the ascending colon and for hepatobiliary surgery. It has the advantages of better cosmesis, less postoperative pain, reduced incidence of postoperative chest infection, and is the preferred incision in children to prevent scar pucker-ing with growth. The disadvantages of this incision include the need to divide muscle, resulting in greater blood loss, and a higher incidence of incisional hernias. In addition, it takes longer to open and close, and cannot easily be extended.

2. Midline laparotomy incisions are quick to open and close, and provide excellent access to most abdominal structures. They are relatively easy to extend, and do not result in significant amounts of blood loss due to the relatively avascular plane involved.

3. McBurney's incision is made over McBurney's point at right angles to a line joining the umbilicus to the anterior superior iliac spine, and was traditionally used as the incision of choice for appendicectomy. In comparison, the Lanz incision is smaller, more transverse, and lies along the skin crease to give a better cosmetic result. The Rutherford Morrison incision is a muscle-splitting incision that may be used for difficult appendicectomies.

23. Answers: 1-F; 2-C; 3-I

1. This patient is highly likely to have developed bony metastasis from his colonic malignancy. Metastatic bone pain is often best controlled by a single dose of fractionated radiotherapy. Bisphosphonates can also be used to reduce osteoclastic activity and non-steroidal anti-inflammatory drugs may be used for their co-analgesic effects.

2. This patient's radiological findings are highly suggestive of metachronous hepatic metastasis from her previous colonic malignancy. Non-steroidal anti-inflammatory drugs and steroids are excellent therapeutic measures for pain caused by the stretching of the liver capsule, due to their ability to decrease swelling and inflammation.

3. This patient demonstrates signs and symptoms of neuropathic pain secondary to probable axillary nodal metastasis from a recurrent breast tumour. Although neuropathic pain is often resistant to simple analgesia, it responds well to anticonvulsants and antidepressants in most patients. For patients whose neuropathic pain is resistant to oral pharmacological therapy, nerve blocks may be attempted to good effect.

24. Answers: 1-B; 2-A; 3-G

The principles of surgery in gastrointestinal perforations are as follows:

- Close the perforation when the underlying disease is likely to heal spontaneously (e.g. perforated peptic ulcer).
- Resect any perforated bowel that is intrinsically diseased. Primary anastomosis should be avoided in the presence of established sepsis, diffuse malignancy, chronic malnutrition, and in significantly ill patients. A stoma should be formed in these circumstances.

1. Perforated gastric ulcers are usually excised before closure due to the associated the risk of malignancy. This may not be possible if the ulcer is very large or suggestive of malignancy. In such cases, the appropriate partial or total gastrectomy should be performed.

2. Perforated duodenal ulcers heal well by closure with an omental patch. A laparotomy including the placement of an omental patch that is secured with sutures, and a thorough peritoneal toilet, is the management of choice. Pre-pyloric ulcers are similar to duodenal ulcers and can be treated in the same way with an omental patch.

3. Large, malignant ulcers in the body of the stomach will necessitate a total gastrectomy with Roux-en-Y reconstruction.

It should be noted that a Billroth I procedure involves a partial gastrectomy with simple re-anastomosis (i.e. gastroduodenostomy); while a Billroth II procedure involves a partial gastrectomy with oversewing of the duodenal stump (thus leaving a blind loop) and anastomosis by a longitudinal incision further down (i.e. gastrojejunostomy). Both Billroth I and II partial gastrectomies can lead to alkaline reflux gastritis, which may be treated with cholestyramine, and occasionally, Roux-en-Y jejunostomy.

1. **Common surgical conditions and the subspecialties: Gastrointestinal disease**

   A. Pilonidal sinus
   B. Pelvirectal abscess
   C. Perianal abscess
   D. Anal fissure
   E. Submucous abscess
   F. Ischiorectal abscess
   G. Fistula-in-ano
   H. Pilonidal abscess

   For each of the following situations, select the single most likely diagnosis from the options listed. Each option may be used once, more than once, or not at all.

   1. A 16-year-old boy presents to the Emergency Department with a 5-day history of progressively worsening pain and swelling in his perianal region. On examination, a tender, cystic lump is seen and felt at the verge of the anal canal, just below the dentate line. The patient's vital signs are normal.

   2. A 35-year-old male presents to the Emergency Department with a 4-day history of peri-rectal pain and feeling generally unwell. Digital rectal examination reveals a tender, indurated swelling over the posterior circumference of the anal canal, above the dentate line. The patient is found to be pyrexial at 39°C, with otherwise normal vital signs.

   3. A 34-year-old female, who is an inpatient in the surgical ward 4 days post-appendicectomy, complains of pain and swelling in her perineal region. She is febrile with a temperature of 38.4°C and is systemically unwell. Digital rectal examination reveals a fluctuant, tender swelling higher up in the rectum, close to the upper surface of the levator ani muscle and the pelvic peritoneum.

2. **Common surgical conditions and the subspecialties: Gastrointestinal disease**

A. Achalasia cardia
B. Barrett's oesophagus
C. Benign oesophageal stricture
D. Bolus impaction
E. Caustic oesophagitis
F. Gastro-oesophageal reflux disease
G. Globus pharyngeus
H. Oesophageal carcinoma
I. Pharyngeal carcinoma
J. Plummer–Vinson syndrome

For each of the following situations, select the single most likely diagnosis from the options listed. Each option may be used once, more than once, or not at all.

1. A 76-year-old female with no significant past medical history presents to her GP with a 3-month history of progressively worsening, burning retrosternal pain. The pain is worse at night and is aggravated by drinking hot liquids. Further questioning reveals a sensation of food 'sticking to the bottom of her gullet'. There is no history of regurgitation of food and no constitutional symptoms.

2. A 74-year-old retired engineer presents to his GP with a 6-month history of progressive dysphagia and weight loss of 9 kg in that period. His dysphagia was initially to solids but he now has difficulty in swallowing tea. He has no other constitutional symptoms and no significant past medical history or family history.

3. A 32-year-old solicitor presents to her GP with a 12-month history of intermittent difficulty in swallowing. She describes dysphagia to both liquids and solids but denies any constitutional symptoms. She has no significant past medical history or relevant family history.

3. **The assessment and management of the surgical patient:**
   Differential diagnosis
   A. Acute appendicitis
   B. Intussusception
   C. Acute pancreatitis
   D. Intestinal obstruction
   E. Diabetes mellitus
   F. Acute intermittent porphyria
   G. Constipation
   H. Mesenteric adenitis
   I. Urinary tract infection

   For each of the following situations, select the single most likely diagnosis from the options listed. Each option may be used once, more than once, or not at all.

   1. A 6-month-old girl presents to the Paediatric Emergency Department with a 12-hour history of episodic screaming, drawing up of her knees, and vomiting. This was preceded by fever and diarrhoea, with the passage of red mucoid stools. Abdominal examination is challenging as the child is restless. What is the most likely cause of her symptoms?

   2. A 7-year-old boy presents to the Paediatric Emergency Department with a 2-day history of abdominal pain, fever, anorexia and nausea. On examination, he is pyrexial at 38.4°C and has lower abdominal tenderness, mainly in the right iliac fossa. What is the most likely cause of his symptoms?

   3. A 9-year-old boy presents to his GP with a 4-day history of feeling unwell, coryza, abdominal pain and vomiting. On examination, he is pyrexial at 39.2°C with vague, generalized lower abdominal tenderness. What is the most likely cause of his symptoms?

4. **Perioperative care: Postoperative complications**
   A. Air leak
   B. Arrhythmia
   C. Atelectasis
   D. Haemorrhage
   E. Bronchopleural fistula
   F. Cardiac failure
   G. Myocardial infarction
   H. Pneumonia

   For each of the following situations, select the single most likely postoperative complication from the options listed. Each option may be used once, more than once, or not at all.

   1. A 58-year-old male undergoes a pneumonectomy for locally advanced lung cancer. On postoperative day 7, he develops sudden breathlessness and expectorates blood-stained sputum. Examination of the chest reveals dullness to percussion on the side of the surgery, and the chest drain appears to be draining blood-stained fluid similar to that coughed up.

   2. A 60-year-old patient undergoes a cardio-oesophagectomy for distal oesophageal cancer. On postoperative day 3, he is found to be tachypnoeic and hypoxic but apyrexial. Examination of the chest reveals decreased bibasal air entry.

   3. A 65-year-old male undergoes a left pneumonectomy for locally advanced lung cancer. In the immediate postoperative period, he is found to be in respiratory distress. Examination reveals a raised JVP and bibasal crepitations. Chest radiography reveals a small bilateral pleural effusions, Kerley B lines and upper lobe diversion.

5. Assessment and management of patients with trauma (including the multiply injured patient): Resuscitation and early management

A. Absolute contraindication for thoracotomy
B. Absolute indication for thoracotomy
C. Relative contraindication for thoracotomy
D. Relative indication for thoracotomy
E. Fluid resuscitation prior to haemorrhage control
F. Chest drain insertion
G. Needle thoracostomy decompression
H. Conservative management
I. None of the above

For each of the following situations, select the single most appropriate intervention, or circumstance, from the options listed. Each option may be used once, more than once, or not at all.

1. A 23-year-old man presents to the Emergency Department after being stabbed in the left side of his chest with an unidentified object. On examination, he is found to be dyspnoeic, tachycardic and hypotensive, with a raised JVP and muffled heart sounds. His ECG reveals small QRS complexes and a FAST scan confirms cardiac tamponade.

2. A 54-year-old male is brought to the Emergency Department in an unconscious state. There were no witnesses at the scene but he is assumed to have sustained blunt trauma to his chest due to the pattern of bruising evident. He undergoes ten minutes of cardiopulmonary resuscitation with no response.

3. A 30-year-old boxer is brought to the Emergency Department after receiving a series of heavy punches to his abdomen. He is found to be hypotensive and tachycardic, and examination of his abdomen reveals generalised tenderness and peritonism. An emergency laparotomy is performed on the basis of a probable intra-abdominal haemorrhage. Intraoperatively, a small hole is found in the aorta, at the level of the renal arteries, from which the surgeon struggles to control the active bleeding.

6. **Basic and applied sciences: Pathology**
   A. ABL
   B. APC
   C. C-erbB-2
   D. C-myc
   E. C-sis
   F. Cyclin kinase
   G. Epidermal-derived growth factor
   H. HER-2
   I. p53
   J. K-ras

   For each of the following descriptions, select the single most likely gene or protein from the options listed. Each option may be used once, more than once, or not at all.

   1. This oncogene fuses with the BCR gene on the Philadelphia chromosome, which is a characteristic abnormality seen in chronic myeloid leukaemia.

   2. This is a tumour suppressor gene which plays important roles in apoptosis, genetic stability, and the inhibition of angiogenesis. It is associated with conditions such as Li–Fraumeni syndrome and cervical cancer.

   3. The translocation of this oncogene with chromosome 8 results in the development of Burkitt's lymphoma.

7. **The assessment and management of the surgical patient: Clinical decision-making**
   A. Non-steroidal anti-inflammatory drugs
   B. Admission and intravenous antibiotics
   C. High-grade compression bandaging
   D. Rest, oral antibiotics and simple analgesics
   E. Rest and elevation
   F. Intravenous heparin
   G. Simple dressings and retention bandaging
   H. Urgent surgery
   I. Oral warfarin

   For each of the following situations, select the single most appropriate treatment from the options listed. Each option may be used once, more than once, or not at all.

   1. A 59-year-old woman with a history of chronic venous insufficiency presents to her GP with a 2-day history of pain and increased exudate from her right leg ulcer. On examination, the area surrounding the ulcer is red, warm and painful. The ankle–brachial pressure index (ABPI) in this leg is 1.02. The patient is otherwise asymptomatic and has a temperature of 37.4°C.

   2. A 53-year-old woman presents to the surgical outpatient clinic with a 12-week history of a left lower leg ulcer. On examination, the ulcer lies over the medial malleolus and has gentle sloping edges. The area surrounding the ulcer appears pigmented. The peripheral pulses are palpable and the ABPI in the affected limb is 1.0.

   3. A 68-year-old man in the orthopaedic ward experiences pain and swelling in his left calf 8 days after undergoing a total hip replacement. On examination, the left calf is swollen, red, tender, and warm to touch. The patient's temperature is 37.8°C and his vital signs are otherwise normal.

8.   Perioperative care: Critical care

A. Adrenaline (intramuscular)
B. Adrenaline (intravenous)
C. Dobutamine
D. Dopamine (large dose)
E. Dopamine (small dose)
F. Dopexamine
G. Isoprenaline
H. Nitrates
I. Noradrenaline

For each of the following situations, select the single most appropriate treatment from the options listed. Each option may be used once, more than once, or not at all.

1. A 55-year-old lady is admitted to the Surgical Assessment Unit with the signs and symptoms of acute diverticulitis. She is prescribed co-amoxiclav, but on administration of this drug, she experiences neck swelling, cyanosis, and drooling of saliva.

2. A 70-year-old lady is admitted to the Surgical Assessment Unit with suggested ascending cholangitis. Despite treatment with intravenous antibiotics and intravenous fluid, she becomes confused, pyrexial with a temperature of 38°C, and tachycardic, with a low urine output. She is transferred to the High Dependency Unit, where she receives arterial and central venous pressure (CVP) lines and aggressive fluid management. Despite such significant efforts, her CVP remains at 8 mmHg, urine output remains under 0.5 mL/hour, and serum lactate remains at over 4 mmol/L.

3. A 58-year-old male undergoes an elective total hip replacement. On postoperative day 1, he becomes cold, clammy, and complains of central crushing chest pain. On examination, his pulse rate is 130/min, BP is 84/50 mmHg, and auscultation of his chest reveals bibasal crepitations and a third heart sound. A 12-lead ECG reveals ST elevation in leads V2–V4. He is treated with high-flow oxygen, morphine and high-dose aspirin, and he undergoes an emergency percutaneous angioplasty. However, he remains hypotensive and tachycardic following this procedure.

9. Professional behaviour and leadership: Medical consent

A. Bolam test
B. Consent form 1
C. Consent form 2
D. Consent form 3
E. Consent form 4
F. Gillick competence
G. Implied consent
H. Proceed under the Mental Capacity Act
I. Verbal consent

For each of the following situations, select the single most appropriate consent-related test, documentation or circumstance, from the options listed. Each option may be used once, more than once, or not at all.

1. A 15-year-old boy presents to the Emergency Department with a 2-hour history of acute scrotal pain and swelling that is highly suggestive of testicular torsion. He is accompanied by his father, although it is his mother who holds parental custody since their divorce. The boy needs to be consented for a scrotal exploration. What circumstance may allow him to consent to his operation?

2. A 60-year-old nursing home resident with severe vascular dementia is brought into the Emergency Department by ambulance, with acute abdominal pain. Examination reveals generalised peritonitis, prompting the need for an emergency laparotomy. Although he is able to communicate, he is disorientated and is unable to retain any information given to him. Two consultants subsequently agree on the management plan and proceed to sign a consent form.

3. A 14-year-old girl presents to the Emergency Department with acute abdominal pain that is highly suggestive of acute appendicitis. After obstetric and gynaecological causes are excluded, the surgeon wishes to proceed with an appendicectomy due the patient's worsening septic signs. Although the patient does not fully understand the benefits and risks involved, she is reluctant to undergo surgery. The patient's mother is therefore approached by the surgeon to sign a consent form on the patient's behalf.

10. **The assessment and management of the surgical patient: Clinical decision-making**

A. Right hemicolectomy
B. Subtotal colectomy
C. Transverse colectomy
D. Abdominoperineal resection
E. Anterior resection
F. Debulking using radiotherapy
G. Extended right hemicolectomy
H. Hartmann's procedure

For each of the following situations, select the single most appropriate operative intervention from the options listed. Each option may be used once, more than once, or not at all.

1. A 63-year-old male is awaiting curative surgery for a localized, non-invasive tumour of the caecum. His past medical history includes only bronchial asthma and hayfever. What will be the most appropriate treatment option for this patient?

2. A 71-year-old female with a history of osteoarthritis and mild hypertension is admitted to the Surgical Assessment Unit for abdominal pain and weight loss. She is subsequently diagnosed with a Dukes B colonic tumour in the region of the hepatic flexure, with no evidence of lymphatic or distant metastasis. What is the most appropriate treatment option for this patient?

3. A 68-year-old male, who is under the care of the colorectal surgeons, is undergoing treatment for a localized tumour in the distal third of his rectum, 3 cm from the anal verge. His past medical history includes only diet-controlled diabetes mellitus. A staging MRI scan of the abdomen and pelvis excludes metastatic disease and reveals that the tumour has advanced through the bowel wall. What is the most appropriate treatment option for this patient?

11. Perioperative care: Assessing and planning nutritional management

A. Jejunostomy feeding
B. Nasoenteric fine-bore feeding
C. Nasogastric tube feeding
D. Oral feeding
E. Percutaneous endoscopic gastrostomy feeding
F. Peripheral parenteral nutrition
G. Special enteral feeding
H. Total parenteral nutrition

For each of the following situations, select the single most appropriate means of nutrition from the options listed. Each option may be used once, more than once, or not at all.

1. A 72-year-old gentleman has recently suffered from an extensive stroke, with residual left-sided hemiparesis, dysphagia and dysarthria. He is due for neurorehabilitation and requires long-term nutritional support.

2. A 19-year-old motorist sustains a moderate head injury from a high-speed road traffic accident, and is admitted to the neurosurgical ward for further assessment. His GCS on admission is 9 but he begins to demonstrate gradual signs of recovery shortly thereafter. The multidisciplinary team discusses the most appropriate means of nutritional support for the patient.

3. A 63-year-old man is diagnosed with stage 2 oesophageal carcinoma, and is awaiting surgery with curative intent. The surgeon wishes to perform the procedure via an Ivor Lewis approach. During preoperative counselling, the surgeon describes the operation to the patient and also highlights the need for additional long-term nutritional support, in view of the patient's weight loss of 25 kg over the previous three months.

12. Professional behaviour and leadership: Medical consent

A. Obtain consent from the child
B. Obtain consent from the parent with legal custody
C. Obtain consent from the step-parent, if a legal custodian is not available
D. Obtain lasting power of attorney
E. Obtain consent from an independent mental capacity advocate
F. Obtain a court order
G. Obtain consent from the senior-most attending clinician
H. Obtain consent from the General Medical Council
I. Obtain consent from the Medical Defence Union
J. Accept the patient's decision against medical advice

For each of the following situations, select the most appropriate course of action from the options listed. Each option may be used once, more than once, or not at all.

1. A 15-year-old boy presents to the Emergency Department with his step-father, complaining of symptoms consistent with acute appendicitis. He is assessed by the consultant surgeon, who feels that an appendicectomy is warranted. The surgeon explains the condition and procedure to the child and finds that he is able to understand and retain the information provided. He is also able to weigh up the risks and benefits of surgery, and agrees to have the operation.

2. A 15-year-old boy presents to the Emergency Department following a road traffic accident. Shortly after a CT scan, which confirms the presence of a shattered spleen, the patient rapidly becomes haemodynamically unstable. Although the patient is formally deemed to have capacity, he refuses the consultant surgeon's strong recommendation to undergo an emergency splenectomy. His parents cannot be contacted during this time.

3. A 15-year-old girl is required to undergo general anaesthesia for the removal of a percutaneous endoscopic gastrostomy tube, as decided by the attending consultant and his colleagues. She is deemed to be competent but refuses the procedure, for no apparent reason. Her mother also refuses to give consent to the procedure on her behalf.

13. The assessment and management of the surgical patient: Clinical decision-making

A. Dynamic Doppler ultrasound imaging of groin
B. Elective exploration of groin
C. Elective hernia repair with mesh fixation
D. Emergency exploration and repair of defect
E. Expedited elective hernia repair with mesh fixation (as a day-case procedure)
F. Expedited elective hernia repair with mesh fixation (as an inpatient procedure)
G. Shouldice hernia repair
H. Truss support
I. Urgent duplex ultrasound imaging

For each of the following situations, select the most appropriate immediate diagnostic or treatment modality from the options listed. Each option may be used once, more than once, or not at all.

1. A 54-year-old male presents to the Emergency Department with colicky abdominal pain and constipation. He has only been passing flatus for the previous 48 hours. Examination reveals a distended, tympanitic and generally tender abdomen, with high-pitched bowel sounds heard on auscultation. An exquisitely tender, firm, irreducible lump is palpable in his right inguinal region.

2. An 88-year-old male with severe COPD and left ventricular hypertrophy presents to his GP with a two-year history of a progressively enlarging, irreducible lump in his inguinal region. It is non-tender, with a positive cough impulse, and no bowel sounds are audible within it.

3. A 75-year-old male with medication-controlled atrial fibrillation, hypertension and insulin-dependent diabetes mellitus, presents to his GP with a gradually enlarging lump immediately above and medial to his right pubic tubercle. On examination, it is non-tender, partially reducible and has a positive cough impulse.

14. Perioperative care: Critical care

A. Compensated metabolic acidosis
B. Compensated respiratory acidosis
C. Metabolic acidosis with normal anion gap
D. Metabolic acidosis with increased anion gap
E. Compensated respiratory alkalosis
F. Compensated metabolic alkalosis
G. Respiratory acidosis
H. Respiratory alkalosis
I. Metabolic alkalosis

For each of the following situations, select the single most likely abnormality in acid–base balance from the options listed. Each option may be used once, more than once, or not at all.

1. An 80-year-old man presents to the Emergency Department with acute, severe epigastric pain. Examination reveals generalised abdominal peritonitis and the results of his arterial blood gas analysis are as follows: pH 7.4, pO_2 12 kPa, pCO_2 3.0 kPa, base excess −8.0 mmol/L, HCO_3 15 mmol/L, Na 132 mmol/L, K 3.0 mmol/L, Cl 95 mmol/L, urea 12.0 mmol/L and creatinine 180 µmol/L. What is the most likely acid–base disturbance?

2. A 68-year-old man with atrial fibrillation presents to the Emergency Department with a 4-hour history of severe, generalized abdominal pain. Examination reveals tachycardia and hypotension with generalized abdominal peritonitis. The results of the arterial blood gas analysis are as follows: pH 7.28, pCO_2 4.0 kPa, pO_2 10.0 kPa, base excess −10 mmol/L, HCO_3 15 mmol/L, Na 136 mmol/L, K 3.0 mmol/L, Cl 96 mmol/L, urea 12.0 mmol/L and creatinine 140 µmol/L. What is the most likely acid–base disturbance?

3. A 56-year-old man undergoes a laparoscopic Nissen fundoplication. In the early postoperative period, he develops shortness of breath and the results of the arterial blood gas analysis are as follows: pH 7.3, pO_2 7.0 kPa, pCO_2 6.6 kPa, HCO_3 26 mmol/L, base excess −2 mmol/L, Na 135 mmol/L, K 3.2 mmol/L, Cl 100 mmol/L, urea 9.0 mmol/L and creatinine 120 µmol/L. What is the most likely acid–base disturbance?

15. The assessment and management of the surgical patient: Planning investigations

A. Alpha-fetoprotein
B. Beta-2 microglobulin
C. Beta-HCG
D. CA 19-9
E. CA 125
F. CA 15–3
G. Calcitonin
H. Chromogranin A
I. Prostate-specific antigen

For each of the following situations, select the serum marker that is most likely to be elevated from the options listed. Each option may be used once, more than once, or not at all.

1. A 54-year-old woman presents to her GP with a 4-month history of progressively worsening flushing and diarrhoea. A thorough physical examination reveals a prominent thyroid nodule at the base of her neck and associated cervical lymphadenopathy.

2. A 40-year-old woman presents to her GP with a 6-month history of intermittent colicky central abdominal pain and diarrhoea. These episodes are associated with flushing, palpitations and occasional dyspnoea.

3. A 65-year-old African man presents with a 12-month history of worsening back pain, generalized muscle weakness and anorexia. Examination reveals limited lumbar spine movement but no evidence of neurological deficit. His laboratory investigations reveal a haemoglobin level of 7.7 g/dL, haematocrit of 23%, platelet count of 10×10^9/L, creatinine of 380 µmol/L, urea of 26 mmol/L and corrected calcium of 3.2 mmol/L. Plain radiography of his spine demonstrates multiple radiolucent foci within the lumbar vertebral bodies.

16. Perioperative care: Assessing and planning nutritional management

A. Enteral feeding via nasojejunal tube

B. High-energy supplement drinks

C. Immune modulating feeds

D. Low residual diet

E. Parenteral feeding

F. Feeding jejunostomy

G. Small bowel follow-through

H. Start erythromycin

I. Terminal ileal biopsy

For each of the following situations, select the single most appropriate initial investigation or management from the options listed. Each option may be used once, more than once, or not at all.

1. A 30-year-old female, who has previously undergone a total pancreatectomy and Roux loop reconstruction, presents to her GP with signs and symptoms of malnutrition despite her normal dietary intake and Creon® supplementation. Her symptoms include chronic abdominal pain, nausea and intermittent vomiting.

2. A 60-year-old female endures a prolonged hospital admission for acute-on-chronic pancreatitis. She is unable to tolerate an oral diet due to persistent nausea and vomiting. Nasogastric tube insertion is unsuccessful due to intractable retching.

3. A 68-year-old man is due to undergo a cardio-oesophagectomy for locally advanced oesophagogastric cancer, followed by a course of adjuvant chemotherapy. His family is keen to know how he is likely to be fed after his operation.

17. The assessment and management of the surgical patient: Differential diagnosis

A. Direct inguinal hernia

B. Encysted hydrocoele

C. Femoral artery aneurysm

D. Femoral hernia

E. Indirect inguinal hernia

F. Inguinal lymphadenopathy

G. Lipoma

H. Obturator hernia

I. Neuroma of femoral nerve

J. Saphena varix

For each of the following situations, select the single most likely diagnosis from the options listed. Each option may be used once, more than once, or not at all.

1. A 5-week-old boy is brought to the GP by his parents, who have noticed a swelling in his left groin. They report that the swelling appears when the child strains or cries, and disappears at rest.

2. A 68-year-old woman presents to the Emergency Department with a 12-hour history of sudden-onset, colicky, central abdominal pain and vomiting. Further questioning reveals that she has not opened her bowels since the previous morning. Examination reveals generalized abdominal tenderness and distension but no signs of peritonism. In addition, an erythematous, exquisitely tender groin lump is noted below and lateral to the pubic tubercle.

3. A 65-year-old gentleman with severe chronic obstructive airways disease presents to his GP with a 2-month history of an asymptomatic swelling in his right groin. Examination reveals a non-tender and reducible lump, above and medial to the public tubercle. After reduction, the lump reappears with coughing, despite pressure over the deep inguinal ring.

18. **Assessment and management of patients with trauma (including the multiply injured patient): History, examination, and investigation**

A. Abdominal radiograph
B. Computed tomography scan
C. Diagnostic peritoneal lavage
D. Erect chest radiograph
E. FAST scan
F. Laparoscopy
G. Laparotomy
H. Ultrasound scan

For each of the following situations, select the single most appropriate initial investigation from the options listed. Each option may be used once, more than once, or not at all.

1. A 60-year-old female is brought to the Emergency Department after having been involved in a road traffic accident. On examination, the patient has an obvious fracture of her right proximal femur, and is found to be haemodynamically unstable. Her abdomen is distended and tender in the right iliac fossa, with no signs of peritonism.

2. A 32-year-old female is involved in a head-on road traffic collision with a truck. On arrival to the Emergency Department, she is found to be haemodynamically stable. Examination of her abdomen reveals significant epigastric and right upper quadrant tenderness but no evidence of peritonism. A CT scan is unable to exclude a diaphragmatic injury.

3. A 13-year-old boy presents to the Emergency Department after falling off a 2-metre climbing frame and landing on his back. He is found to have sustained fractures to three right lower posterior ribs. Tenderness and bruising is evident over his right loin, and a urine specimen is observed to have macroscopic haematuria.

19. The assessment and management of the surgical patient: Clinical decision-making

A. Endoscopic mucosal resection
B. Endoscopic sclerotherapy
C. Heller's cardiomyotomy
D. Ivor Lewis procedure
E. Nissen fundoplication
F. Oesophageal balloon dilation
G. Oesophagogastrectomy
H. Oesophagojejunostomy
I. Sengstaken–Blakemore tube placement
J. Transhiatal oesophagectomy

For each of the following situations, select the single most appropriate surgical procedure from the options listed. Each option may be used once, more than once, or not at all.

1. A 39-year-old bank manager presents to her GP with an 18-month history of progressively worsening heartburn. This has occurred despite her having lost weight, stopping smoking, and taking maximum antisecretory medication as prescribed. An oesophagogastroduodenscopy (OGD) reveals no abnormalities but 24-hour oesophageal pH monitoring confirms GORD.

2. A 75-year-old retired solicitor is referred by his GP to the upper GI surgeons for a 6-month history of worsening dysphagia, anaemia, and unexplained weight loss. An OGD confirms an oesophageal tumour at 32 cm, and a staging CT scan confirms paraoesophageal lymph node involvement.

3. A 57-year-old businesswoman is referred by her GP to the surgical outpatient department for a 3-month history of worsening dysphagia. She has not lost any weight and is systemically well. However, an OGD and biopsy confirm distal oesophageal adenocarcinoma. A staging CT and endoscopic ultrasound suggest no local invasion or lymphatic involvement.

20. Surgical care of the paediatric patient: History, examination, and assessment of neonates and children

A. Meconium ileus

B. Duodenal atresia

C. Anorectal atresia

D. Volvulus neonatorum

E. Tracheo-oesophageal fistula

F. Intussusception

G. Congenital hypertrophic pyloric stenosis

H. Hirschsprung's disease

I. Necrotizing enterocolitis

For each of the following situations, select the single most likely diagnosis from the options listed. Each option may be used once, more than once, or not at all.

1. A 5-day-old baby girl with cystic fibrosis is brought to the Emergency Department with gross abdominal distension and bilious vomiting. She is not taking regular feeds and appears dehydrated. Plain abdominal radiography reveals distended coils of bowel but no overt fluid levels.

2. A 31-week-old baby boy (born prematurely) in the paediatric ward is asked to be reviewed with a distended and tense abdomen. The baby is passing blood and mucus per rectum. She is also manifesting signs of sepsis. Plain abdominal radiography reveals distended loops of bowel and gas bubbles within the bowel wall.

3. A 3-day-old baby boy is brought to the Emergency Department with mild abdominal distension and failure to pass meconium after birth. The child is crying constantly. Barium enema reveals the descending colon to have a narrow segment associated with a dilated proximal colon.

21. The assessment and management of the surgical patient: Appropriate prescribing

A. Aminoglutethimide
B. Androgen receptor antagonist (e.g. cyproterone acetate) and goserelin
C. Aromatase inhibitor (e.g. anastrozole)
D. Gonadotropin-releasing hormone agonist (goserelin)
E. Medroxyprogesterone
F. Oestrogen agonist (e.g. diethylstilbestrol)
G. Oestrogen hormone replacement
H. Oestrogen receptor antagonist (e.g. tamoxifen)
I. Somatostatin analogue (e.g. octreotide)

For each of the following situations, select the single most appropriate hormone therapy from the options listed. Each option may be used once, more than once, or not at all.

1. A 65-year-old postmenopausal female has recently been diagnosed with oestrogen receptor-positive breast cancer. The multidisciplinary team decides to commence her on adjuvant hormonal therapy following the surgical clearance of her tumour.

2. A 67-year-old male is referred by his GP to the Urologists with a 2-month history of progressively worsening obstructive urological symptoms, bone pains and weight loss. Clinical examination reveals a hard, irregularly enlarged prostate gland; and subsequent imaging tests confirm the diagnosis of metastatic prostate cancer.

3. A 60-year-old who female, who has undergone a abdominal hysterectomy and bilateral salpingo-oophorectomy for well-differentiated, early endometrial adenocarcinoma, presents to her GP with signs and symptoms of tumour recurrence. Urgent investigations confirm the late malignant spread of her cancer to the pelvis (i.e. stage III disease).

22. Basic surgical skills: Surgical technique

A. Lembert suture technique
B. Modified Kessler suture technique
C. Whiting's manoeuvre
D. Jaboulay's technique
E. Halstead suture technique
F. Pringle manoeuvre
G. Karydakis technique
H. Z-plasty technique
I. Lord's plication

For each of the following situations, select the single most appropriate surgical technique from the options listed. Each option may be used once, more than once, or not at all.

1. A 3-month-old baby undergoes Ramstedt's procedure for hypertrophic pyloric stenosis. Which surgical technique is used to reduce the risk of perforation during this procedure?

2. A 30-year-old man is scheduled for surgery to repair the complete laceration of a flexor tendon in his hand. Which surgical technique is best used for this operation?

3. A 24-year-old man is referred by his GP to the colorectal surgeons with a 4-week history of intermittent discharge and discomfort in his natal cleft. He has previously undergone two drainage procedures for pilonidal sinuses in that region. He is now diagnosed with a chronic pilonidal sinus and is scheduled for surgery. Which surgical technique is best used for this operation?

23. **Assessment and management of patients with trauma (including the multiply injured patient): Assessment, scoring, and triage of adults and children**

A. Debride wound, reduce fracture, close wound and splint
B. Debride wound, reduce fracture, externally fix and close wound
C. Debride wound, reduce fracture, externally fix and leave wound open
D. Debride wound, reduce fracture, internally fix and close wound
E. Debride wound, reduce fracture, internally fix and leave wound open
F. Debride wound, reduce fracture, splint and leave wound open
G. Reduce fracture, internally fix and close wound
H. Reduce fracture and apply backslab
I. Reduce fracture and apply cylindrical plaster

For each of the following situations, select the single most appropriate sequence of interventions from the options listed. Each option may be used once, more than once, or not at all.

1. A 16-year-old female presents to the Emergency Department following a fall during a gymnastic performance. Examination reveals no open wounds but there is significant swelling and tenderness over her left distal tibia. A plain radiograph of the limb confirms an oblique fracture of the distal tibia with no involvement of the ankle joint. The patient has no collateral injuries and is haemodynamically stable.

2. A 40-year-old farmer sustains injuries to his lower leg from being trapped under a tractor in a field. He presents to the Emergency Department 7 hours after the injury, and is found to have a 10 cm open wound and a deformed leg that maintains its neurovascular integrity. Plain radiography of the limb reveals a significantly angulated, minimally translated, transverse, mid-shaft fracture of the tibia. The patient has no collateral injuries and is haemodynamically stable.

3. A 20-year-old cyclist is brought to the Emergency Department after being hit by a car travelling at 50 miles/hour. The primary survey is normal and any head or neck injuries are excluded. The secondary survey reveals a 5 cm open wound, with comminuted tibial fracture involving exposed bone and extensive soft tissue damage. The patient has no collateral injuries and is haemodynamically stable.

24. Basic surgical skills: Use of drains

A. Blake drain

B. Corrugated drain

C. Foley catheter

D. Multi-holed polyvinyl chloride drain

E. Penrose drain

F. Pigtail drain

G. Redivac drain

H. Robinson drain

I. T-tube

For each of the following situations, select the single most appropriate type of drain from the options listed. Each option may be used once, more than once, or not at all.

1. A 45-year-old patient undergoes a Hartmann's procedure for a perforated sigmoid diverticulum. Throughout the operation, the gross intraperitoneal contamination is thoroughly washed out with copious amounts of warm saline, and a drain is inserted towards the end of the procedure.

2. A 55-year-old male undergoes an elective mesh repair of a large incisional hernia. Due to the extensive tissue dissection undertaken during the procedure, a drain is inserted towards the end, to prevent haematoma formation.

3. A 35-year-old female undergoes a laparoscopic cholecystectomy and common bile duct exploration for the retrieval of a large common bile duct stone. The procedure is technically challenging, and is complicated by the inadvertent formation of a small hole in the posterior aspect of the common bile duct, and failure to retrieve the stone. The surgeon decides to insert a drain into the common bile duct to minimize bile leakage and facilitate healing.

1. Answers: 1-C; 2-F; 3-B

Perirectal abscesses comprise perianal abscesses (60%, immediately adjacent to the anal verge); ischiorectal abscesses (25%, inferior to the levator ani and 2–3 cm from the anal verge); pelvirectal abscesses (superior to the levator ani, and originating from a pelvic or intra-abdominal source); and intersphincteric abscesses.

1. Perianal abscesses may occur in patients of all ages, including infants and children. The constitutional symptoms and localized pain are less pronounced than in ischiorectal abscesses because the pus can expand the walls of this aspect of the intermuscular space comparatively easily. Early diagnosis can be made by inspecting the anal margin, when an acutely tender, rounded, cystic lump (usually about the size of cherry) may be seen and felt. In some cases, rigid sigmoidoscopy may be necessary to find the perianal abscess outlet. Pus should be sent for culture of both routine gut and skin organisms, and additionally, acid fast bacilli. Specimens of the abscess should be sent for histopathological examination. When detection occurs early, treatment with oral antibiotics may abort the infection. In cases of established infection, drainage and curettage (i.e. usually performed under general anaesthesia) may be required. The patient may remain in hospital for 3–7 days and be off work for 1–4 weeks.

2. Ischiorectal abscesses more commonly affect men than women. Patients may present with features of systemic upset, with high pyrexia (e.g. temperatures of 39–40°C). An ischiorectal abscess initially gives rise to a tender, brawny induration along the affected side of the anal canal, above the dentate line. The ischiorectal fossa communicates with that of the opposite side via the post-sphincteric space so if an ischiorectal abscess is not evacuated early, the contralateral fossa is soon involved. This may result in a 'horseshoe' abscess, which envelopes the whole of the posterior part of the circumference of anal canal. The management of ischiorectal abscess is similar to that of perianal abscess, with incision and drainage forming the mainstay of definitive treatment.

3. A pelvirectal abscess is a recognized complication of appendicectomy. This may either result from a perforated appendix or peritoneal contamination and infection following appendicectomy. A pelvirectal abscess is situated between the upper surface of the levator ani and pelvic peritoneum. Crohn's disease, pelvic inflammatory disease and diverticulitis are other recognized causes of pelvirectal abscesses. As with other forms of perirectal abscesses, surgical drainage forms the mainstay of treatment for pelvirectal abscesses.

2. Answers: 1-C; 2-H; 3-A

Dysphagia is defined as difficulty in swallowing, in contrast to odynophagia, which refers to painful deglutition. As with various other tubal pathologies, dysphagia may be due to intraluminal, mural (i.e. including muscular disorders), extrinsic, or functional causes. The symptom of dysphagia may be described by some patients as a 'sticking' sensation, the site of which is usually well localized, especially in the upper two-thirds of the oesophagus, which has a predominantly somatic rather than visceral innervation.

1. A retrosternal burning sensation is most characteristic of GORD. It may be aggravated by ingesting food or drink (especially if hot). The fact that this is associated with 'stickiness' of food in this patient is suggestive of a stricture. The lack of systemic symptoms (e.g. anorexia, weight loss, lethargy) goes against the suggestion of malignancy, although this must always be definitively excluded in elderly patients. Although this patient may certainly harbour a degree of metaplastic change (i.e. Barrett's oesophagus), this alone is unlikely to cause mechanical obstruction of food to give dysphagia.

Such benign peptic strictures are a result of chronic injury to the oesophagus by gastric acid, or more rarely, bile. They occur in 15% of patients with reflux oesophagitis, and tend to occur at the distal squamocolumnar junction; the majority are less than 2 cm in length. Histologically, strictures show submucosal fibrosis, destruction of the muscularis mucosae, and varying amounts of perioesophageal inflammatory change. As mentioned, it is vital to differentiate this from malignancy (i.e. with barium swallow, followed by endoscopy). Management may be conservative (e.g. with proton pump inhibitors, which are highly effective; or endoscopic balloon dilatation) or surgical (resection of the affected segment with colonic interposition).

2. The cause of dysphagia in this elderly gentleman is likely to be malignancy due to its insidious progression, the patient's age and his significant weight loss. The incidence of oesophageal carcinoma (especially of the gastro-oesophageal junction) has been rising, unlike that of gastric cancer. It is strongly linked to alcohol (especially spirits) and smoking. The principle symptom is dysphagia, and physical signs are rare apart from wasting (and perhaps the finding of Virchow's node). Patients can often localize the level of the obstruction in their oesophagus fairly accurately (e.g. carcinoma of the distal oesophagus may be described as a blocked sensation behind the lower end of the sternum).

Following history and examination, the diagnostic workup includes barium swallow, endoscopy and biopsy, CT (or MRI), bronchoscopy, and ultrasonography (i.e. transoesophageal ultrasound if possible). Staging is vital to prevent unnecessary surgical intervention, and may involve the earlier described investigations and diagnostic laparoscopy.

The management of oesophageal carcinoma depends on the level of the lesion and the stage of the disease. For proximal lesions, high-dose radiotherapy is indicated for lesions up to 5 cm long. Surgical clearance is challenging in this area due to vital structures in the adjacent mediastinum. For lesions in the middle third, radical radiotherapy may be used for lesions up to 5 cm long; early tumours here are resectable. Lesions in the distal third can usually be accessed surgically (note: adenocarcinomas, which most commonly occur here, are largely radioresistant). Advanced or metastatic disease that is not amenable to surgery requires palliation of the dysphagia. This may be achieved by endoscopic laser ablation (for lesions <8 cm long), oesophageal stenting, gastrostomy- or jejunostomy-feeding, or short-course radiotherapy.

3. The long history of intermittent dysphagia (to both solids and liquids equally) and lack of other symptoms in this previous well lady suggests achalasia as the problem. This rare condition (annual incidence 1 per 100,000) involves the neuromuscular failure of relaxation of the distal oesophagus, with progressive dilatation, tortuosity, incoordination of peristalsis, and often hypertrophy of the proximal segment. This effectively results in a functional obstruction at the distal oesophagus. It usually manifests in the 3rd to 4th decades, and presents equally commonly in males and females. Due to the neuromuscular aetiology of achalasia, the dysphagia tends not to present as progressively as it does with benign or malignant strictures.

Investigations include barium swallow, which demonstrates the characteristic 'bird's beak' appearance with proximal dilatation and distal smooth tapering; and endoscopy, to exclude malignancy and other pathologies. Chest radiography may reveal a widened mediastinum with a fluid level behind the cardiac shadow, and the absence of a gastric air bubble. Manometric studies reveal only partially relaxation of the distal gastro-oesophageal sphincter, with a high resting tone that does not fall to gastric fundal pressure.

Although achalasia is considered to be incurable, relief of the distal obstruction (and hence the dysphagia) may be achieved by the following means:

- Pharmacological: intrasphincteric botulinum toxin injection, especially for patients with idiopathic achalasia who are at high risk of complications of pneumatic dilatation or surgical myotomy.
- Endoscopic: hydrostatic or pneumatic dilatation, which may be repeated monthly. Although dilatation has a low mortality, oesophageal perforation may occur in 2% of cases.
- Surgical: Heller's cardiomyotomy, which involves an incision in the distal 3–4 cm of oesophageal muscle longitudinally. The success rate of this is about 90% in those who do not respond to dilatation.

It is important to note that both the endoscopic and surgical treatments may result in reflux oesophagitis. Overall, the complications of achalasia include aspiration pneumonia, haemorrhage and oesophageal carcinoma.

3. Answers: 1-B; 2-A; 3-H

1. Intussusception refers to the invagination of one portion of bowel into the lumen of the immediately adjoining bowel. The most common form is the result of an origin in terminal ileum or the ileo-caecal valve resulting in an ileocolic intussusception. It has a peak incidence at 3–7 months of age, and is usually associated with a prodromal illness, often with diarrhoea. Early symptoms include paroxysms of colicky abdominal pain lasting a few minutes. Vomiting becomes bilious and more frequent as intestinal obstruction develops. Late symptoms include mucoid, bloody 'red currant jelly' stools suggestive of intestinal ischaemia. A palpable abdominal mass in the right upper quadrant (Dance's sign) may be found on examination. Abdominal ultrasonography is the gold standard for diagnosis, on which intussusception is recognized by the presence of the 'target' or 'sandwich' sign. The treatment of choice involves reduction by barium enema (or an air enema) under radiological control. However, a barium enema is contraindicated if there are features of perforation or generalized peritonitis. Indications for surgery include clinical signs of peritonitis, gross dehydration, failure of medical treatment or recurrence thereafter, and children aged under 3 months or over 2 years.

2 and 3. Mesenteric adenitis is the commonest imitator of appendicitis in children. Its peak incidence is in prepubertal children and it is uncommon after 15 years of age. Mesenteric adenitis is usually caused by viral or, less commonly, bacterial infection of mesenteric lymph nodes. Preceding viral upper respiratory tract infections with high fever, malaise, headache, sore throat and cough are commonly observed in mesenteric adenitis. In contrast, appendicitis usually has a fairly rapid onset with progressive deterioration.

The abdominal pain experienced in mesenteric adenitis is usually diffuse, central and colicky. Appendicitis may initially present in this way as well, but tends to deteriorate and localize to the right iliac fossa, with signs of peritonism. While anorexia is a feature of both conditions, appendicitis is more commonly associated with nausea and vomiting. In addition, examination of the ears, nose, and throat may be normal in appendicitis, but usually reveals cervical lymphadenopathy with or without an erythematous upper respiratory tract, in mesenteric adenitis.

4. Answers: 1-E; 2-C; 3-F

1. Bronchopulmonary fistulae complicate approximately 2% of pneumonectomies. They result from the breakdown of the suture line of the bronchial stump and subsequent air leakage.

The airway is thus in direct communication with the pleural space. This usually occurs 7–10 days following surgery and presents with the patient expectorating blood-stained fluid, which is usually found in the post-pneumonectomy space. The emergency management of such patients consists of laying the patient flat (i.e. with the operated side downwards), oxygenation, and drainage of the pleural space with a surgical chest drain. In patients with a persisting fistula, thoracotomy and repair of the fistula with an omental or intercostal muscle flap may be necessary. Thoracoplasty may also be performed to obliterate the intercostal space.

2. Postoperative pain following a thoracotomy restrains deep breathing and the clearing of bronchial secretions. This causes bronchial obstruction, atelectasis, lobar collapse, and secondary pulmonary infection. The risk of atelectasis may be reduced by preoperative cessation of smoking, adequate postoperative pain relief, chest physiotherapy, humidified oxygen usage, bronchodilation, and early mobilization following surgery. Antibiotics should only be used in patients with confirmed chest infection. Although atelectasis would be the commonest cause for tachypnoea and hypoxia in such patients after major surgery, it is imperative that postoperative pulmonary embolism is clinically excluded (i.e. with D-dimer measurement and subsequent imaging, if necessary).

3. Pneumonectomy involves the removal of a significant part of the pulmonary circulation. Such a decrease in pulmonary vascular volume may result in an increase in the pulmonary vascular resistance, thereby precipitating right heart failure. This may be confirmed clinically, with the aid of chest radiography (i.e. demonstrating a 'bat-wing' pattern of alveolar oedema; interstitial oedema marked by Kerley B lines; cardiomegaly; upper lobe blood diversion; and pleural effusions). In the acute setting, this may be managed with supplemental oxygenation, diuresis (e.g. with furosemide) and drugs inducing vasodilatation (e.g. morphine and glyceryl trinitrate), followed by urgent senior medical review.

5. Answers: 1-B; 2-A; 3-D

1. This scenario describes cardiac tamponade following a penetrating chest injury, which is an absolute indication for emergency thoracotomy. Other absolute indications include:

- Traumatic arrest following penetrating thoracic injury with previously witnessed cardiac activity (i.e. pre-hospital or in-hospital)
- An unresponsive, hypotensive patient with a penetrating thoracic injury
- An unresponsive, hypotensive patient who has sustained a blunt thoracic injury
- Rapid exsanguination from a chest drain of >1500 mL of blood

2. There are five specific contraindications to emergency thoracotomy:

- Blunt chest trauma with absence of signs of life
- CPR for more than 10 minutes after blunt trauma
- CPR for more than 5 minutes without endotracheal intubation
- No spontaneous cardiac electrical activity for more than 10 minutes
- Severe head injury

Although emergency thoracotomy is indicated for internal cardiac massage in cases with massive exsanguination from chest drains, it should not be performed as an alternative to closed massage or chest compressions unless there are other clinical reasons to do so.

3. In situations such as this, with massive intra-abdominal haemorrhage, a thoracotomy may be performed in order to achieve proximal control of the haemorrhage by cross-clamping the thoracic aorta. This will improve the cardiac and cerebral circulation and give the surgeon a clearer field and adequate time to deal with the intra-abdominal trauma.

Other relative indications for an emergency thoracotomy include:

- Traumatic arrest with penetrating thoracic injury without previously witnessed cardiac activity
- Traumatic arrest following blunt thoracic injury in a patient with previously witnessed cardiac activity.

6. Answers: 1-A; 2-I; 3-D

Normal genes involved in cell division are called proto-oncogenes. These genes become permanently activated by point mutation, translocation or amplification. These genes code for growth factors, receptors, signal transducing proteins and transcription factors. Therefore, upregulation of these genes results in uncontrolled cell division and growth.

1. When the ABL (Abelson murine leukaemia viral oncogene homolog 1) proto-oncogene found on chromosome 9 is translocated with the breakpoint cluster (BCR) gene on chromosome 22, it becomes activated and encodes for the production of tyrosine kinase, which allows cells to proliferate without cytokine-driven regulation. This subsequently results in a clonal myeloproliferative disorder.

2. p53 is known as the guardian of the genome as it plays an important role in control of the cell cycle and apoptosis. DNA damage by mutagens increases the amount of p53, which has three major functions: growth arrest, DNA repair and apoptosis. The growth arrest stops the progression of the cell cycle, preventing the replication of damaged DNA. During the growth arrest, p53 may activate the transcription of proteins involved in DNA repair. Apoptosis is the 'last resort' to avoid proliferation of cells containing abnormal DNA. The concentration of p53 within a cell is tightly regulated by MDM2, which can trigger the degradation of p53 by the ubiquitin system.

The mutation of p53 results in abnormal cell proliferation and cancer—approximately 50% of all cancers contain mutated p53 genes.

Li–Fraumeni syndrome is an autosomal dominant hereditary disorder that results from a germ-line mutation of the p53 gene. People with this syndrome have an increased risk of developing breast cancer, brain tumours, acute leukaemia, soft tissue sarcomas, bone sarcoma and adrenal carcinomas.

3. The translocation of the c-myc gene between chromosomes 8 and 14 is involved in the development of Burkett's lymphoma. This translocation activates c-myc to produce transcription factors that are involved in gene amplification, presumably through DNA replication.

7. Answers: 1-D; 2-C; 3-F

1. This patient has developed cellulitis, probably from her infected venous ulcer. Due to the early presentation and the fact that the patient remains systemically well, the most appropriate treatment at this stage would be rest, oral antibiotics (usually flucloxacillin, against *Staphylococcus aureus*), and simple analgesia. If there is greenish exudate or malodour from the ulcer, infection due to *Pseudomonas aeruginosa* may be suspected and this should be treated with a quinolone derivative such as ciprofloxacin.

2. This is a classical presentation of a simple venous leg ulcer. Such ulcers are usually located over the 'gaiter region' (i.e. on the medial aspect of the leg, between the medial malleolus and the knee) and have gently sloping edges. Since there is adequate arterial circulation with a normal ABPI, the most appropriate treatment would be high-grade compression bandaging. This may be in the form of elastic or inelastic compression bandages or tubular bandages (e.g. Tubigrip®).

3. This patient is very likely to have developed a postoperative DVT. This is classically seen 7–10 days after surgery. Patients typically experience pain and swelling in the affected leg (calf). Examination may reveal a warm, red, tender calf with an increase in the calf girth. Serum D-dimer measurements and Duplex ultrasound scanning may be necessary to confirm or exclude the diagnosis. Upon confirmation of a DVT, treatment should be commenced with intravenous heparin followed by treatment with oral warfarin.

8. Answers: 1-A; 2-I; 3-C

1. This scenario describes a case of drug-induced anaphylaxis. As with all emergency scenarios, this patient should first be resuscitated using the 'ABC' approach. In addition, 0.5 mL of 1:1000 adrenaline should immediately be administered intramuscularly. This may be repeated as necessary at 5-minute intervals. Patients should also receive antihistamines, intravenous hydrocortisone and intravenous fluids to maintain their blood pressure. The adrenaline serves to act on α receptors, causing peripheral vasoconstriction, and causes positive chronotropia by acting on β1 receptors. By therefore increasing systemic vascular resistance and cardiac output, it acts to normalise the blood pressure. Moreover, adrenaline also acts on β2 receptors of the lungs, causing bronchodilatation and immediate symptomatic relief to the anaphylactic patient.

2. This patient is profoundly septic with her circulating inflammatory mediators causing extensive peripheral vasodilatation. Noradrenaline acts primarily on α receptors to cause peripheral arterial and venous vasoconstriction, thereby increasing systemic vascular resistance. It should be administered centrally—in low doses, only an arterial line or central venous line may be adequate, but at higher doses, a Swan-Ganz catheter is required. The rise in systemic vascular resistance induced by noradrenaline is an effective way of managing refractory sepsis-related hypotension but must be done so in an appropriate environment (e.g. within the Intensive Care Unit or High Dependency Unit).

3. This scenario describes cardiogenic shock following a postoperative myocardial infarction. The cardiac muscle is unable to contract efficiently enough to eject the end-diastolic volume. The cardiac stroke volume falls and as a consequence, the body responds as if it is dealing with hypovolaemia, by peripheral vasoconstriction and fluid retention. Dobutamine is a synthetic form of isoprenaline and acts predominantly on β1 receptors, increasing the force of myocardial contraction, and to a smaller extent on β2 receptors, to offload the heart. As with noradrenaline, this drug should be administered under strict monitoring, although it may be given through a peripheral venous line if a central line is not immediately available.

9. Answers: 1-F; 2-E; 3-C

1. In this scenario, the father of the boy is unable to consent for the operation as he has no legal parental custody over the child. Although the child is aged less than 16 years, he may be deemed to possess sufficient mental capacity to understand what is proposed, retain the information and weigh the pros against the cons. The child may therefore be deemed as Gillick competent by the senior clinician in charge of his care, and may be permitted to consent to some procedures but not for others – this remains at the discretion of the responsible clinician.

2. This patient is unable to retain the given information for long enough to weigh up the pros and cons in the decision-making process. He is therefore deemed to be incompetent to give consent to treatment. None of the patient's friends or relatives will be able to give or withhold consent for any procedure on his behalf. After having considered such factors, the clinician in charge of the patient's care is expected to act in the patient's best interest. Such professional judgement should stand up to the Bolam test and therefore the consent form 4 (i.e. for adults

who do not have the capacity to consent) should be signed by two clinicians, in order for treatment to proceed.

3. For children under the age of 16 years, who are considered to be 'Gillick incompetent', consent may be obtained from the parents or legal guardian, using consent form 2. This is especially applicable for patients requiring urgent or emergent surgery for life-threatening (or limb-threatening) conditions, where further time cannot be wasted to allow the incompetent patient to comprehend, weigh up and reiterate the pros and cons of treatment.

10. Answers: 1-A; 2-G; 3-D

1. Tumours of the caecum and the ascending colon, which are amenable to surgery, are treated primarily by means of a right hemicolectomy and ligation of the ileocolic and right colic vascular pedicles. The right hemicolectomy involves a resection of the terminal segment of the ileum, caecum, ascending colon and the right half of the transverse colon, along with the corresponding mesentery.

2. The most appropriate surgical procedure for this patient is the extended right hemicolectomy. Since the transverse colectomy is associated with a high rate of anastomotic leakage, tumours of the proximal transverse colon such as those in the hepatic flexure are treated by means of an extended right hemicolectomy. In this procedure, the bowel is divided proximally at the terminal ileum and distally across the descending/sigmoid colon. The ends of the bowel are then anastomosed either using staples or using a hand-sewn technique. In the extended right hemicolectomy, the ileocolic artery, right colic artery and middle colic artery (with or without the ascending branch of the left colic artery) are ligated and divided.

3. Rectal malignancy that has advanced through the bowel wall requires radical excision of the tumour along with the surrounding affected tissue. Total mesorectal excision in conjunction with a low anterior resection or abdominoperineal resection is the optimal treatment for mid-rectal and low-rectal tumours that have advanced locally. This technique involves the removal of the entire rectal mesentery to 5 cm below the tumour. The patient in this scenario will require an abdominoperineal resection (with total mesorectal excision) due to the proximity of his tumour to the anal verge.

11. Answers: Answers: 1-E; 2-B; 3-A

Nutritional support should be administered enterally, whenever possible, as this decreases the incidence of peptic ulceration and hepatorenal dysfunction, reduces the incidence of bacterial translocation from the gut, and reduces the risk of line-related and stoma-related complications.

1. Percutaneous endoscopic gastrostomy (PEG) feeding should be considered for patients who cannot meet their nutritional requirements orally, and require nutritional support for at least 4 weeks. Examples of such circumstances include:

- Neurological dysphagia with potential for recovery from the underlying disease (e.g. multiple acute strokes); or when recovery is unlikely (e.g. motor neuron disease)
- Inability to eat due to global neurological damage, with potential for recovery from the underlying disease (e.g. reversible brain injury); or without potential for recovery (e.g. comatose state, severe stroke, severe dementia, etc.)
- Mechanical dysphagia due to obstruction to the proximal upper GI tract (e.g. head and neck cancer)
- Inability to cope with anorexia or increased catabolism from chronic disease states (e.g. chronic renal failure); or malabsorption syndromes such as cystic fibrosis and Crohn's disease
- Psychiatric disorders causing refusal to eat (e.g. depression or anorexia nervosa)

2. Nasoenteric (or 'nasoduodenal') tubes are fine-bore weighted tubes passed into the duodenum via the nose, which are used for short- or medium-term nutritional support. These tubes are particularly indicated in patients with abnormal pyloric function, problems with aspiration, or in patients with delayed gastric emptying. Since this patient is recovering from a head injury (i.e. potentially involving a degree of neurological dysphagia and delayed gastric emptying), nasoenteric fine-bore feeding is the most appropriate means of short-term nutritional support for him.

3. In the two-stage Ivor Lewis (or 'Lewis–Tanner') oesophagectomy procedure, the patient undergoes an initial laparotomy and construction of a gastric tube, followed by a right thoracotomy to excise the tumour (together with perioesophageal tissue, including lymph nodes) and create an oesophagogastric anastomosis. To provide nutritional support in view of his significant recent weight loss (which is probably attributable to a combination of dysphagia and malignancy), a perioperative feeding jejunostomy may be fashioned. Two other common approaches to oesophagectomy include the thoracoabdominal approach (i.e. opening the abdominal and thoracic cavities together); and the three-stage McKeown approach (i.e. involving a third incision in the neck to complete the cervical anastomosis).

12. Answers: 1-A; 2-G; 3-J

1. All children under the age of 16 years are able to give consent to a procedure, treatment or investigation if they are deemed to be Gillick competent. This child is considered to be Gillick competent as he is able to understand, retain, and weigh up the pros and cons of the information that he has been provided with. Therefore, despite the absence of his legal custodian, he should be allowed to give consent for his own treatment. It should be noted that even if this child was not Gillick competent, consent should not be obtained from his step-father, who does not have the legal right to provide it.

2. In the emergency setting, the clinician is obliged to provide emergency treatment (i.e. with or without consent) to save the life of, or to prevent further deterioration in the health of, a child or young person. The child's parents should be involved in the process wherever possible but treatment should not be delayed until consent is received from them or the courts. If the parents disagree, the clinician is entitled to proceed with whatever is perceived to be in the best interest of the child.

3. In either the elective or emergency setting, a child who is deemed to be Gillick competent should be allowed to give or refuse consent to his or her treatment. If the child was incompetent and treatment was deemed essential (or in the best interests of the patient), and the accompanying parent or legal guardian refused to give consent, a court order may be sought. However, in this case, there is no urgency or other indication to overrule the competent patient's decision.

13. Answers: 1-D; 2-H; 3-F

Despite the fact that most inguinal hernias are benign and asymptomatic, it is imperative that clinicians are able to identify their complications, and to have a low threshold for acting on hernias that may be incarcerated, obstructed or strangulated. Amongst inguinal hernias, indirect hernias (80%) are significantly more common than direct hernias (20%). Due to their course via the deep ring into the inguinal canal, indirect hernias have a much higher risk of incarceration and strangulation, whereas direct hernias (which occur through a weakness in the transversalis fascia) reduce easily, and therefore rarely strangulate. In contrast to inguinal hernias, femoral hernias (which typically occur in elderly females) are frequently irreducible and frequently strangulate, due to the narrow neck of the femoral canal.

1. The pain and tenderness described in this scenario are highly suggestive of bowel obstruction secondary to a strangulated inguinal hernia. If this persists for much longer, there is a risk of ischaemia to the loop of bowel trapped within the hernia sac, and subsequent systemic toxicity. Such a presentation therefore warrants an emergency operation to release and fix the hernia.

2. This scenario highlights the importance of being able to recognize which patients are appropriate candidates for surgery. This elderly patient's multiple comorbidities place him at a high anaesthetic and surgical risk for any procedure. His minimally symptomatic hernia pathology may therefore be best managed conservatively, with a supportive truss device.

3. As this patient's hernia is only partially reducible, it is incarcerated and requires prompt elective repair to minimize any future risk of obstruction or strangulation. Given the history of atrial fibrillation, he is likely to be on warfarin therapy, which will need stopping prior to the operation, as well as postoperative reloading, making him a suitable candidate for an inpatient procedure.

14. Answers: 1-A; 2-D; 3-G

The normal ranges of arterial blood gas components (i.e. measured at body temperature, and while inspiring room air) are as follows:

- pH: 7.35–7.45
- pO_2: 10–13.3 kPa
- pCO_2: 4.6–6 kPa
- HCO_3: 22–26 mmol/L
- Base excess: −2.4 to +2.2 mmol/L
- Arterial O_2 saturation: 95–98%
- Mixed venous oxygen saturation: 70–75%.

A pH of <7.35 indicates acidosis and a pH of >7.45 indicates alkalosis. In cases of metabolic acidosis, an understanding of the anion gap may help to determine the cause of the acidosis. The anion gap is the difference between the measured cations and the measure anions, which can be estimated by: Anion gap = $(Na + K) − (Cl + HCO_3)$, the normal range for which is 10–18 mmol/L. The anion gap helps to differentiate between those causes of acidosis that occur due to loss of bicarbonate and those that occur due to increased levels of organic acid. A 'normal anion gap' metabolic acidosis may be observed in profuse diarrhoea, renal tubular acidosis, Addison's disease, pancreatic fistulae, ammonium chloride ingestion and by certain drugs (e.g. acetazolamide). A 'high anion gap' metabolic acidosis may be observed in cases of lactic acidosis (e.g. shock, sepsis, hypoxia), uraemia (e.g. renal failure), ketosis (e.g. diabetes mellitus, alcohol intoxication), and by certain drugs (e.g. aspirin, metformin, ethylene glycol, methanol).

Respiratory acidosis occurs due to excess CO_2 production and/or inadequate excretion (e.g. hypoventilation, excess narcotic usage). Respiratory alkalosis is frequently due to a reduction in pCO_2 due to hyperventilation. Metabolic alkalosis may be due to excessive vomiting, potassium depletion (e.g. from diuretics), burns or ingestion of alkaline material.

1. Although this patient has a primary metabolic acidosis of a probable intra-abdominal cause, his respiratory buffer is able to compensate for this (i.e. respiratory compensation) to ensure that his pH remains within the normal range. This is termed 'compensated metabolic acidosis'.

2. This patient is acidotic, with a low bicarbonate (i.e. metabolic acidosis), and a raised anion gap: $(Na + K) − (Cl + HCO_3) = (136 + 3.0) − (96 + 15) = 28$ mmol/L. This is probably due to a rise in serum lactate secondary to ongoing mesenteric ischaemia.

3. This patient has developed type 2 respiratory failure (i.e. with a low pO_2 and high pCO_2). One may assume that this has not yet been fully compensated for (i.e. pH 7.3) by the kidneys, which need time to increase the serum HCO_3 to do so. As the pH has yet to normalise, this is simply considered as uncompensated respiratory acidosis.

15. Answers: 1-G; 2-H; 3-B

1. Medullary thyroid carcinoma arises from the thyroid parafollicular cells (C cells), which are responsible for the production of calcitonin. About 25% of these tumours are familial and result from a mutation of the RET proto-oncogene. The others may be sporadic or associated with phaeochromocytomas and parathyroid tumours in the MEN 2 (multiple endocrine neoplasia type 2) syndrome. Medullary thyroid carcinoma can metastasize to lymph nodes, liver, lung and bones. The mainstay of treatment for this type of thyroid malignancy includes surgery and external beam radiotherapy.

2. Carcinoid tumours are neuroendocrine tumours derived from the primitive neural crest. They are most commonly found in the midgut (i.e. appendix 45%, ileum 30%, rectum 20%) and arise from enterochromaffin cells. Only about 10% of these secrete excessive amounts of hormones, such as serotonin. Carcinoid syndrome implies hepatic involvement (5% of carcinoid tumours), causing symptoms of flushing, diarrhoea, abdominal pains, wheezing, and peripheral oedema (secondary to CCF from serotonin-induced tricuspid incontinence and pulmonary stenosis). If carcinoid is suspected, the diagnostic workup should include blood tests for chromogranin A, fasting plasma 5-hydroxyindoleacetic acid (HIAA) levels, urinary 5-HIAA levels and an octreotide scan. Chromogranin A levels are elevated in 80–100% of carcinoid tumours and are useful in their detection and monitoring. The management of carcinoid syndrome involves octreotide (i.e. to block the release of tumour mediators and counter peripheral effects) and interferon-α. Tumour therapy involves surgical debulking, embolization of radiofrequency ablation of hepatic metastases.

3. This clinical picture of anaemia, thrombocytopenia, renal insufficiency, hypercalcaemia, and multiple lytic bone lesions in an elderly patient is strongly suggestive of multiple myeloma. This is a disease characterized by the malignant proliferation of plasma cells and the overproduction of monoclonal paraproteins. The diagnosis itself is made by measuring serum calcium and ESR, plasma electrophoresis (demonstrating monoclonal IgG bands), and the finding of urinary Bence-Jones proteins and plasma cells on bone marrow biopsy. Treatment comprises supportive therapy (e.g. focusing on the bone pathology, anaemia, renal impairment and prophylaxis against infections) and chemotherapy. Median survival is poor at 3-4 years. Beta-2 microglobulin is a marker of overall body tumour burden and a strong prognostic indicator of outcome (i.e. it is associated with a worse prognosis).

16. Answers: 1-G; 2-E; 3-F

1 Although chronic pain is expected in patients following pancreatectomy, severe nausea and vomiting frequently indicate intestinal obstruction. Given this patient's past surgical history, blind loop syndrome must be considered. Blind loop syndrome occurs when there is an obstructed or bypassed portion of intestine. This segment is deprived of digestive juices and bile, resulting in impaired fat digestion and steatorrhoea. The stagnant food ferments, creating an ideal environment for bacterial overgrowth. These bacteria interfere with absorption of nutrients and vitamins which often lead to weight loss and malnutrition.

2. Intolerance of nasogastric feeding precludes enteral feeding in this patient, leaving parenteral feeding to be the only option. Parenteral nutrition may be administered either via central or

peripheral venous access. In 10% of these patients, line-related complications may develop, including sepsis. It is imperative that biochemical markers be monitored (e.g. serum phosphate, to monitor for refeeding syndrome). A major disadvantage of parenteral nutrition compared to enteral nutrition is the risk of intestinal mucosal atrophy, followed by an increased risk of bacterial translocation across the gut wall, leading to SIRS and multiple organ dysfunction syndrome.

3. Patients who undergo an oesophagectomy (e.g. for gastro-oesophageal malignancy) often experience dysphagia and the various side-effects from chemotherapy, including anorexia and weight loss. Patients are often kept nil by mouth for 5–7 days postoperatively to allow for healing of the anastomosis between the oesophagus and the newly fashioned conduit. The placement of a feeding jejunostomy intraoperatively will provide enteral access for these patients, who will experience challenges with oral feeding, and a slow transition back to a normal diet.

17. Answers: 1-E; 2-D; 3-A

When listing the differential diagnosis of groin lumps, it may be helpful to recall pathologies in a 'medial to lateral' manner: hydrocoele or varicocoele, inguinal hernia, femoral hernia, lymph node, saphena varix, femoral artery aneurysm, neuroma of the femoral nerve, and psoas abscess. An undescended testis (i.e. cryptorchidism) is also possible. In addition, intradermal (e.g. sebaceous cyst, abscess, dermoid cyst, granuloma) and subcutaneous (e.g. lipoma, neuroma, ganglion, lymph node) lesions should be considered.

1. A congenital inguinal hernia results from a patent processus vaginalis, and is the commonest indication for surgery in infancy and childhood. The processus vaginalis, which is normally obliterated at around 32 weeks of gestation, may occasionally persist and extend as a hollow tube or sac of peritoneum that extends from the external ring towards the external genitalia. If the opening is narrow, it allows only peritoneal fluid to track down and manifest as a hydrocoele. If the opening is large, various organs (e.g. bowel) may descend along this pathway (i.e. constituting a hernia). The factors causing obliteration of the sac are unknown.

2. Such congenital inguinal hernias occur in 2% of full-term infants and 10% of preterm infants. The male to female ratio is 10:1, with the right side being affected twice as often as the left. It usually present in the first few months of life as a bulge in the groin when the baby cries or strains, which disappears at rest. Most paediatric surgeons practise taxis (i.e. reduction under sedation), followed by herniotomy soon after.

This woman's signs and symptoms are highly suggestive of a strangulated femoral hernia. In comparison to inguinal hernias, which manifest as lumps above and medial to the pubic tubercle, femoral hernias present below and lateral to the pubic tubercle. The anatomy of the narrow femoral canal also makes femoral hernias much more likely to incarcerate, and subsequently strangulate, than inguinal hernias. They also tend to present more commonly in elderly women, as in this case.

Strangulated hernias typically present with signs of intestinal obstruction: colicky abdominal pain, distension, vomiting, and constipation. Localizing symptoms are often absent and there is more discomfort in the abdominal region than in the femoral area. In 30% of cases, a Richter's hernia (i.e. only part of the bowel circumference is trapped in the hernia sac) occurs. Although this tends not to lead to bowel obstruction, the trapped knuckle of bowel may become ischaemic and even perforate into the hernia sac and, subsequently, into the peritoneal cavity.

The management of femoral hernias involves urgent surgical repair (i.e. even of asymptomatic hernias) due to the risk of strangulation of abdominal contents in the canal. The use of a truss is considered dangerous due to its fitting difficulty and the increased risk of strangulation of the contents. Immediate reduction of the hernia clinically is only advisable as a temporary measure, whilst preparations for surgery are made. The operative approach may be abdominal, suprapu-bic, or extraperitoneal; inguinal ('high'); crural ('low'); or transperitoneal. Nevertheless, all meth-ods aim to reduce (or excise) the hernia sac, and reinforce the femoral canal.

3. Unlike indirect inguinal hernias that pass 'indirectly' through the deep inguinal ring, direct inguinal hernias protrude 'directly' forwards through the weakened posterior wall of the inguinal canal (i.e. the transversalis fascia). Direct inguinal hernias occur within the inguinal triangle ('Hesselbach's triangle'), which is bounded medially by the lateral border of the rectus sheath (i.e. the linea semilunaris), superolaterally by the inferior epigastric vessels, and inferiorly by the inguinal ligament. Therefore, the neck of an indirect hernia lies laterally to the inferior epigastric vessels while a direct hernia emerges medial to these vessels. Due to aetiological factors, indirect hernias (75%, including the congenital variants) tend to occur at any age, whilst direct hernias (25%) tend to occur in middle-aged and elderly patients, as the posterior abdominal wall weak-ens. Direct hernias rarely strangulate and tend to be more easily reducible than indirect hernias.

18. Answers: 1-E; 2-G; 3-B

1. Focused assessment with sonography for trauma (FAST) scanning is a four-view mode of ultrasound imaging that can be used to detect as little as 100–250 mL of free fluid within the peri-cardium, and most dependent zones within the peritoneum. It is 86–90% sensitive when com-pared with other modalities of imaging, and is indicated in patients with blunt trauma, whether they are haemodynamically stable or not. In haemodynamically unstable patients, who are too unstable to undergo a CT (i.e. such as the one described in this scenario), a negative FAST scan should prompt a search for other sites of blood loss, or potential causes of non-haemorrhagic shock. A positive FAST scan may warrant a laparotomy in unstable patients.

2. Although this patient remains haemodynamically stable, she demonstrates clear evidence of symptomatic pathology. In view of her equivocal imaging results thus far, diagnostic laparoscopy should be considered at an early stage. Diagnostic laparoscopy has been increasingly used in patients who have sustained abdominal trauma but who are haemodynamically stable and show no indications for urgent laparotomy. It can be used to identify peritoneal perforations and diaphragmatic injuries, and is particularly useful in patients who remain symptomatic despite a negative CT scan.

3. The history (i.e. fall and fracture pattern) and examination findings of this patient are highly suggestive of retroperitoneal haemorrhage secondary to traumatic injury to his right kidney. An intravenous pyelogram would traditionally have been performed to exclude any renal trauma or bladder rupture. In current practice, a contrast CT with angiography (i.e. to assess renal per-fusion) would be the investigation of choice. Early intervention is recommended in the presence of a non-functioning kidney for haemorrhage control and renal salvage. This is becoming increas-ingly feasible in the acute setting due to the wide availability of CT imaging services in Emergency Departments.

19. Answers: 1-E; 2-J; 3-D

1. This patient's history and investigative findings confirm the presence of GORD. Although the first-line (and most sensitive) investigation for suspected GORD is upper GI endoscopy, 24-hour oesophageal pH monitoring may be indicated to confirm intractable GORD if endoscopy findings are normal. Antireflux surgery is indicated for intractable oesophagitis, failure of medical therapy, and complications of GORD (e.g. Barrett's oesophagus). The most common antireflux proce-dure is the laparoscopic Nissen fundoplication, which involves wrapping the gastric fundus 270° around the distal oesophagus, while the latter contains a large-bore NG tube (i.e. to prevent the

wrap from being sutured too tightly). The wrap functions as a 'flutter valve', reducing transient lower oesophageal sphincter relaxation and increasing the angle of oesophageal insertion.

Contraindications to antireflux surgery include prior vagotomy or partial gastrectomy, challenging anatomy (e.g. an enlarged left hepatic lobe, which reduces the laparoscopic field of view), and oesophageal shortening. Potential complications include iatrogenic organ injury, pneumothorax, and 'gas bloat syndrome' due to excessive oesophageal constriction.

2. Provided that this patient is fit for surgery, the treatment of choice would be a transhiatal oesophagectomy. The reason for such an approach would be that the tumour is locally advanced, as demonstrated by the staging CT. In addition, the transhiatal approach is most appropriate for tumours in the upper or lower third of the oesophagus. The operation is performed through a neck incision and laparotomy. The benefit of this approach is that it avoids a thoracotomy and therefore tends to be better tolerated by less fit patients. However, an important disadvantage is that it involves blind dissection around the carina.

3. The history and investigative findings have confirmed an early, distal oesophageal tumour in this patient. The curative procedure of choice would be an Ivor Lewis oesophagectomy, which is a two-stage procedure involving a right thoracotomy and a laparotomy, Such access makes it most suitable for tumours of the middle and lower thirds of the oesophagus. The advantage of this procedure is the excellent exposure and ease of anastomosis. However, the thoracotomy aspect adds considerably to the major morbidity of the procedure. As with any major surgery, careful preoperative workup and patient preference must be taken into consideration to preserve quality of life as much as possible, considering the already poor prognosis of oesophageal malignancy.

20. Answers: 1-A; 2-I; 3-H

1. Meconium ileus affects 1 in 15,000 newborns. This condition is caused by a distal small bowel obstruction secondary to abnormal bulky and viscid meconium. Meconium ileus presents during the first days of life with gross abdominal distension and bilious vomiting. Abnormal meconium is the result of deficient intestinal secretions and 90% of these infants will have cystic fibrosis. Abdominal radiography shows a typical mottled ground-glass appearance due to lipid droplets within the meconium; this has been referred to as a 'soap bubble' appearance, and is usually observed in the right iliac fossa. The bowel distal to the obstruction is usually of small calibre, despite being part of the colon. Fluid levels are scarce as the meconium is viscid in nature. The obstruction may be relieved in uncomplicated cases (e.g. without perforation, volvulus, or atresia) by the administration of one or more enemas with a dilute radiographic contrast medium, plus N-acetylcysteine, under fluoroscopy. Note that the hypertonic contrast material may cause large gastrointestinal water losses, requiring intravenous rehydration. If the enema does not relieve the obstruction, laparotomy may be required. A double-barrelled ileostomy with repeated N-acetylcysteine lavage of the proximal and distal loops is usually required to liquefy and remove the abnormal meconium.

2. Mesenteric ischaemia, resulting from hypoperfusion of the bowel, is more common in premature infants than in full-term infants. The terminal ileum, caecum and distal colon are most commonly affected by this condition. As the degree of ischaemia progresses, intestinal necrosis facilitates bacterial invasion of the gut mucosa (i.e. necrotizing enterocolitis). The affected infant presents with a distended, tense abdomen, and may pass blood and mucus per rectum. Abdominal radiography reveals distended loops of intestine, and gas bubbles may be seen within the bowel wall—'pneumatosis intestinalis'. The management of necrotizing enterocolitis is multimodal, including supportive therapy for immediate complications such as circulatory shock or other disturbances. Oral feeding is stopped for at least a week, with total parenteral

nutrition given over the period of starvation. Feeding is then resumed with caution, using human milk wherever possible. Intravenous broad spectrum antibiotics are administered, and surgical resection may be necessary for necrotic or perforated bowel. Regular girth measurement and serum FBC analysis are helpful in monitoring progress of the acutely unwell child. Abdominal radiology should only be repeated when necessary (e.g. if the child shows evidence of clinical deterioration).

3. Hirschsprung's disease affects 1 in 5000 live births (male: female = 4:1). The pathology involves an absence of ganglion cells in the parasympathetic plexuses of Auerbach and Meissner within the intestinal wall, commencing at the internal anal sphincter and progressing proximally for variable distances. Some affected individuals seem to exhibit an autosomal dominant inheritance; nonetheless, 75% of cases are confined to the rectosigmoid, while 10% of cases involve the entire large bowel. Infants typically present with delayed passage of meconium together with increasing abdominal distension and vomiting, although the condition may rarely present as chronic constipation in infancy. Plain abdominal radiography may reveal signs of intestinal obstruction, while a barium enema may reveal a contracted rectum with a cone-shaped transitional zone and proximal dilatation. Anorectal manometry demonstrates an absence of the normal anorectal inhibitory reflex on rectal distension. The definitive diagnosis is made on rectal biopsy, which demonstrates an absence of submucosal ganglion cells, increased acetylcholinesterase cells in the muscularis mucosa, and an increase of unmyelinated nerves in bowel wall. The initial management involves a defunctioning stoma to relieve the obstruction and reduce the risk of enterocolitis/perforation. Definitive surgery, performed at 6–9 months of age, involves the excision of the aganglionic segment and subsequent anastomosis to the anal canal (Swenson procedure), if possible. Postoperative complications (e.g. constipation, incontinence and diarrhoea) occur in 6–12% of patients.

21. Answers: 1-C; 2-B; 3-E

1. Current NICE guidelines suggest that all postmenopausal patients with oestrogen receptor-positive early invasive breast cancer should be offered adjuvant hormonal therapy with aromatase inhibitors. Adjuvant therapy is given after surgical clearance of all macroscopic disease, in an attempt to destroy microscopic disease and prevent recurrence. Aromatase inhibitors, such as anastrozole, inhibit the production of oestrogen in the peripheral tissues. It is not the first choice of adjuvant treatment in premenopausal women, as the ovaries are the main site of oestrogen production in this age group. The effect of aromatase inhibitors on the hypothalamic–pituitary axis may lead to the overproduction of gonadotropins and hyperstimulation of the ovaries to produce oestrogen, in these younger patients.

2. Hormonal therapy for prostate cancer aims to inhibit the proliferation of malignant prostate cells by androgen deprivation. Approximately 70–80% of these cancers respond to medical androgen ablation. Goserelin is a luteinizing-hormone-releasing-hormone analogue (LHRH), which decreases the synthesis and release of gonadotropins. Within the first fortnight of commencing treatment, it increases LHRH levels, thereby inducing a rapid rise in testosterone, which transiently worsens symptoms and increases prostate specific antigen levels. Therefore, an anti-androgen such as cyproterone acetate should be started prior to goserelin, in order to minimize these circumstances.

3. The primary treatment of early endometrial cancer (i.e. stage I disease – well-differentiated, superficially invasive) is by total abdominal hysterectomy and bilateral salpingo-oophorectomy. High-risk stage I disease (i.e. poorly differentiated, deeply invasive) and stage II disease (i.e. with cervical involvement) are treated similarly but with additional post-operative radiotherapy to

reduce the risk of local recurrence from 20 to 5%. Stage III disease (i.e. with pelvic involvement) and stage IV disease (i.e. with distal metastasis) are typically treated with progestogens such as medroxyprogesterone acetate or megestrol. Chemotherapy may occasionally be used in metastatic disease. The prognosis of endometrial carcinoma is determined by the stage, grade, myometrial invasion and lymph node involvement of the tumour.

22. Answers: 1-C; 2-B; 3-G

1. Ramstedt's pyloromyotomy is the procedure of choice for infantile hypertrophic pyloric stenosis. After the child is placed under general anaesthesia, and gastric lavage is performed under continuous nasogastric aspiration, an incision is made in the right upper quadrant to allow adequate access to the pylorus. A longitudinal serosal incision is made at the hypertrophied pyloroduodenal muscle as far as the mucosa, which is left intact and is seen bulging into the incision. During this procedure, the high risk of perforation at the pyloroduodenal junction may be reduced by invaginating the duodenal mucosa (i.e. Whiting's manoeuvre). It should be noted that postoperative feeding may begin after three hours, initially with glucose-water, followed by 3-hourly milk feeds.

2. This patient has sustained a complete laceration to a flexor tendon in the hand, which requires early and meticulous correction in order to maximize the functional and aesthetic outcomes of treatment. The modified Kessler technique is a commonly used method of correcting tendon injuries. This technique involves the use of two continuous, modified Kessler sutures (i.e. four-strand technique) being placed using 3/0 or 4/0 non-absorbable monofilament sutures. The strength of the repair is considered to be related to the number of suture strands linking the proximal and distal tendon fragments.

3. The Karydakis flap technique, which is used in the treatment of chronic or recurrent pilonidal sinuses, aims to flatten the natal cleft and maintain the midline scar. This entails a deep excision of the affected tissue with stepped excision of natal cleft tissue, mobilization of both medial buttock skin flaps, followed by a sutured closure. It produces good results in expert hands, and failure rates as low as 5%.

Techniques appropriate for the initial presentation of pilonidal sinus include excision and healing by secondary intention, which requires regular wound dressing and shaving, and produces 70–90% healing at 70 days (despite a 5–15% recurrence rate). Excision and primary closure results in 70% healing at 2 weeks but with an expected 20% risk of wound infection. Lord's procedure involves the excision of pits, removal of hair and brushing of tracts, and results in 80–90% healing. In addition, phenol injections (60–70% healing) may be attempted.

23. Answers: 1-G; 2-F; 3-C

The Gustilo–Anderson system is widely used for classifying open fractures. It considers the amount of energy involved, the extent of soft tissue damage, and the degree of wound contamination to determine fracture severity. Type I fractures result from low-energy trauma and involve a wound of less than 1 cm in length. Type II fractures also result from low-energy trauma but these comprise wounds greater than 1 cm in length, with more extensive soft tissue damage. The most severe grade is type III, which results from high-energy trauma and involves extensive soft tissue damage and contamination. Type III injuries are subdivided into three categories: type IIIA, comprising a segmental or severely comminuted open fracture but with adequate soft tissue to cover the bone; type IIIB, involving periosteal stripping and bone exposure (thus needing soft tissue cover); and type IIIC, involving vascular injury requiring repair (regardless of soft tissue injury). Therefore, the progression from grade I to IIIC involves a higher degree of energy towards the injury, greater soft tissue and bone damage, and a higher potential for complications.

1. Most closed tibial fractures can be managed initially in a long leg plaster. If the fracture is closed, there is minimal risk of infection and therefore surgical treatment with internal fixation may be considered. Plates may be inserted via limited dissection to act as an internal splint to protect leg length, angulation and rotation, until the fracture heals by callous formation. The most devastating complication with this procedure is deep sepsis. Reamed or un-reamed intramedullary nails may also be used for internal fixation. These have the added advantage of increased axial weight-bearing and the ability to insert them at a point away from the injury site.

2. This patient has presented with a Gustilo type II fracture, which, due to the absence of concurrent soft tissue injuries, is amenable to wound debridement, fracture reduction and split immobilization. The size and mechanism of injury deem it more appropriate for healing by secondary intention and so the wound should be left open until an appropriate time. It should be noted that patients presenting with open wounds should be given intravenous antibiotics and a tetanus booster if required. The wound should be photographed, swabbed and covered. Patients should be taken to theatre for debridement of wounds and fracture stabilization as soon as possible. If this is delayed by more than 8 hours, these fractures should be treated as Gustilo type III fractures, as they then carry a similar risk of infection.

3. This patient has presented with a Gustilo type IIIB fracture, which, without the need for complex vascular reconstruction, is amenable to wound debridement, fracture reduction and external fixation. Although grade I and II fractures can essentially be treated as closed fractures, grade III injuries are most safely treated with external fixators. External fixators may be utilized to manipulate and stabilize the fracture with no soft tissue dissection at the site of the injury. Any postoperative misalignment may be corrected with simple adjustments rather than reoperation, and the risk of deep sepsis is less than that with plates. As noted earlier, primary closure is avoided (i.e. the wound is left open) due to the underlying risk of infection.

24. Answers: 1-H; 2-G; 3-I

Drains are widely used in surgery for a multitude of reasons: to prevent the accumulation of fluid (e.g. blood, pus and other contaminants) or air (e.g. dead space); and to characterize fluid (e.g. for early identification of anastomotic leakage, etc.)

Drains may be classified as follows:

- *Open or Closed*: Open drains (e.g. corrugated rubber or plastic sheets) drain fluid onto gauze pads or into stoma bags, and are therefore associated with an increased risk of infection. Closed drained (e.g. chest drains, abdominal drains) are formed by tubes draining into bags or bottles, and carry a lower risk of infection.
- *Active or Passive*: Active drains are maintained under low- or high-pressure suction. Passive drains simply function according to differential pressures between the body cavities and the exterior.
- *Silastic or Rubber*: Silastic drains are relatively inert and therefore induce minimal tissue reaction. In contrast, red rubber drains may induce an intense tissue reaction, sometimes purposefully allowing a tract to form (e.g. biliary T-tubes).

1. A Robinson drain is an example of a closed, passive (non-suction) drain that works under the influence of gravity. In this scenario, it is used to exteriorize potential collections of fluid from the wound. Other examples of closed, non-suction drains are: T-tubes, Foley catheters, chest drains and Blake drains.

2. A Redivac drain is a closed suction drain that in this case, is used to minimize dead space and to drain any potential fluid collections. As described above, closed drains minimize the risk of introducing infection, whilst active (suction) drains provide better drainage and encourage earlier wound closure, but may damage adjacent structures.

3. A T-tube is a closed, non-suction drain that in this case, is inserted to divert bile away from the obstruction and to minimize bile leakage into the abdominal cavity. Corrugated and Penrose drains are examples of open, non-suction drains that are frequently used to drain infected fluids.

1. Common surgical conditions and the subspecialties: Skin, head, and neck

A. Stucco keratosis
B. Linear epidermal naevus
C. Sebaceous cyst
D. Lupus vulgaris
E. Dermoid cyst
F. Basal cell carcinoma
G. Seborrhoeic keratosis
H. Xanthelasma
I. Squamous cell carcinoma
J. Dermatofibroma

For each of the following situations, select the single most likely diagnosis from the options listed. Each option may be used once, more than once, or not at all.

1. A 31-year-old lady presents to her GP with a 6-day history of an itchy, painless lesion on her right lower leg. She states that she noticed this lesion following an insect bite 5 days ago whilst she was gardening. Examination reveals a nodular, pigmented lesion that is firm but non-tender, and is freely mobile.

2. A 27-year-old woman of Asian origin presents to her GP with a 6-week history of mild, generalized facial swelling associated with lesions over her face and inside her mouth. She describes anorexia and weight loss, together with feeling unusually tired and feverish in the evenings. Examination reveals multiple, cutaneous, jelly-like nodular lesions over her face. The skin surrounding the lesions appears congested. A few similar lesions are noted within her oral mucosa.

3. A 21-year-old woman presents to her GP with a 6-week history of painful swelling over the nape of her neck. Examination reveals an inflamed, tender, cystic swelling with a central punctum. The patient describes previously having had similar lesions in that region.

4. A 71-year-old farmer is referred by his GP to the Plastic Surgery outpatient clinic with multiple, raised facial lesions. The patient does not seem particularly concerned about the lesion due to their existence for many years. Examination reveals multiple brown, non-tender facial lesions that feel 'greasy' on palpation. Similar lesions are noted over the patient's upper back. Systemic examination is unremarkable and there is no locoregional lymphadenopathy.

2. **Common surgical conditions and the subspecialties: Gastrointestinal disease**

A. Colorectal malignancy
B. Diverticulitis
C. Gastroenteritis
D. Enteral nutrition
E. Malabsorption
F. Radiation enteritis
G. Tropical sprue
H. Ulcerative colitis
I. Zollinger–Ellison syndrome

For each of the following situations, select the single most likely cause of diarrhoea from the options listed. Each option may be used once, more than once, or not at all.

1. A 34-year-old woman presents to her GP with a 3-month history of intermittent, colicky abdominal pain associated with blood and mucus per rectum. Examination of her abdomen reveals moderate tenderness to palpation in the left iliac fossa. She remains haemodynamically stable and afebrile throughout the consultation.

2. A 59-year-old mother-of-three presents to her GP with a 4-week history of intermittent, diffuse abdominal pain and profuse diarrhoea, lethargy and malaise. Her past medical history includes a recent total abdominal hysterectomy, bilateral salpingo-oophorectomy and omentectomy. Examination reveals a dehydrated patient and a diffusely tender abdomen. The patient is haemodynamically stable and afebrile.

3. A 65-year-old man on the general surgical ward develops diarrhoea on day 7 after a pylorus-preserving pancreaticoduodenectomy, whilst receiving nutrition via a feeding jejunostomy. Although pseudomembranous colitis is initially suspected as a result of postoperative antibiotic therapy, a stool culture subsequently excludes this diagnosis.

3. **The assessment and management of the surgical patient: Appropriate prescribing**

A. Flucloxacillin
B. Erythromycin
C. Vancomycin
D. Metronidazole
E. Ciprofloxacin
F. Linezolid
G. Imipenem
H. Tetracycline
I. Gentamicin
J. Trimethoprim
K. Tazocin

For each of the following situations, select the single most appropriate antibiotic therapy from the options listed. Each option may be used once, more than once, or not at all.

1. A 20-year-old woman presents to the surgical assessment unit with right-sided loin pain, diffuse lower abdominal pain and fever. Her vital signs demonstrate a temperature of 39°C and tachycardia. Abdominal examination reveals severe right loin tenderness, moderate suprapubic tenderness and no signs of peritonism. Initial blood tests reveal a Hb level of 12.5 g/dL, platelet count of 425 x 10^9/L, WCC of 24 x 10^9/L, neutrophil count of 18 x 10^9/L and CRP level of 195 mg/L.

2. An 80-year-old man undergoes an emergency laparotomy and subtotal colectomy (with ileostomy) for a caecal perforation secondary to an obstructing sigmoid tumour. During his postoperative recovery on the Intensive Care Unit, he is slow to be weaned off the ventilator. On postoperative day 4, he develops signs and symptoms of pneumonia. His sputum culture subsequently suggests an infection with *Acinetobacter baumannii*.

3. A 25-year-old woman develops a painful, red and swollen right breast, 4 days after the normal vaginal delivery of her child. Examination reveals a 5 x 5 cm superficial, tender, fluctuant mass above the nipple-areolar complex of her right breast, with erythematous overlying skin. Her vital signs show that she is haemodynamically stable and afebrile. Despite having the diagnosis of breast abscess explained to her, she is not keen to have the abscess drained due to her needle phobia.

4. **Perioperative care: Critical care**

    A. Bilevel positive airway pressure ventilation

    B. Controlled mandatory ventilation

    C. Continuous positive airway pressure ventilation

    D. Inverse ratio ventilation

    E. Pressure-controlled ventilation

    F. Positive end-expiratory pressure ventilation

    G. Prone ventilation

    H. Pressure support ventilation

    I. Ventilation on rotating bed

    For each of the following situations involving a patient with ARDS, select the single most appropriate method of ventilation from the options listed. Each option may be used once, more than once, or not at all.

    1. This method of ventilation may be used for spontaneously breathing patients in the early stages of ARDS. It may be administered via nasal cannulas or a face mask, and maintains an airway pressure of 5–10 cmH$_2$O.

    2. This method of ventilation generates a characteristic square pressure waveform, thus optimizing the mean arterial wedge pressure without increasing pulmonary artery wedge pressure.

    3. This method of ventilation prolongs the inspiration to expiration ratio, thus optimizing the mean arterial wedge pressure to improve oxygenation for any given pulmonary artery wedge pressure. However, this may lead to hypercapnoea.

5. **Assessment and management of patients with trauma (including the multiply injured patient): Assessment, scoring, and triage of adults and children**

   A. Basal skull fracture
   B. Subarachnoid haemorrhage
   C. Extradural haematoma
   D. Diffuse axonal injury
   E. Cerebral contusion
   F. Subdural haematoma
   G. Cranial vault fracture
   H. Scalp haematoma
   I. Maxillary fracture

   For each of the following situations, select the single most likely diagnosis from the options listed. Each option may be used once, more than once, or not at all.

   1. A 23-year-old man presents to the Emergency Department after being hit on the head by a cricket ball and collapsing thereafter. His colleague, who was with him throughout the accident, describes him as having lost consciousness for only a few seconds, before regaining consciousness and feeling fine afterwards. While in the Emergency Department, the patient's GCS drops and he gets increasingly confused.

   2. A 30-year-old man is brought to the Emergency Department after being assaulted on the head with a baseball bat. On examination, the patient is unconscious, with right periorbital bruising and bleeding from his nostrils and right ear.

   3. A 70-year-old nursing home resident is brought to the Emergency Department with fluctuating levels of consciousness. His carer claims that he sustained a fall and hit his head on the edge of the bed about 10 days ago. Although the patient describes intermittent headaches since his fall, his gait has suddenly become unsteady over the past 2 days. His past medical history includes hypertension and atrial fibrillation.

6. Basic and applied sciences: Microbiology

A. *Staphylococcus aureus*
B. *Streptococcus pyogenes*
C. *Pneumocystis jirovecii*
D. *Mycobacterium tuberculosis*
E. *Pseudomonas aeruginosa*
F. *Escherichia coli*
G. *Clostridium difficile*
H. *Bacteroides fragilis*
I. *Clostridium perfringens*
J. *Candida albicans*

For each of the following situations, select the single most likely causative organism from the options listed. Each option may be used once, more than once, or not at all.

1. A 10-year-old boy is brought to the GP by his parents with a 3-day history of a burning, itching sensation, and redness of his cheeks. He has experienced fever, malaise, and chills and mentions that he has recently recovered from a throat infection. Examination reveals erythema, induration, and tenderness of both cheeks with palpable cervical lymphadenopathy.

2. A 30-year-old woman presents to her GP with a 9-day history of pain in her right breast associated with reddening around the right nipple-areolar complex, and intermittent purulent nipple discharge. Examination reveals generalised right breast tenderness with peri-areolar inflammation, but no evident lumps on palpation.

3. A 60-year-old man undergoes a right hemicolectomy for a Dukes A caecal tumour. He develops signs of pneumonia on postoperative day 4, and is started on a course of antibiotics. Three days after this, he begins to develop abdominal pain, fever and profuse diarrhoea.

7. The assessment and management of the surgical patient: Surgical history and examination

A. Injury to the upper cord of brachial plexus
B. Posterior interosseous nerve lesion
C. Injury to the radial nerve at the level of the axilla
D. Injury to the lower cord of brachial plexus
E. Injury to the radial nerve at the level of the mid-shaft of humerus
F. Anterior interosseous nerve lesion
G. Injury to the radial nerve at the level of the wrist
H. Ulnar nerve injury
I. Median nerve compression

For each of the following situations, select the single most likely diagnosis from the options listed. Each option may be used once, more than once, or not at all.

1. A 20-year-old man is brought to the Emergency Department with a painful arm and an inability to use his left hand, after being involved in a high-speed motorcycle accident. On examination, there is weakness of the wrist with an inability to extend the wrist or fingers of the left hand. There is also loss of extension at the left elbow joint, loss of the left triceps reflex, and sensory impairment over the dorsum of the left forearm.

2. A 31-year-old man presents to the Emergency Department with a deep laceration over the volar surface of his left lower forearm, after being slashed with broken glass during a fight. On examination, he is unable to spread his fingers or to grip a pen firmly. In addition, paraesthesia is noted over the little and ring fingers of the affected side.

3. A 59-year-old woman presents to the Emergency Department after falling on her outstretched hand, with an inability to extend the metacarpophalangeal joints of her right hand, and wrist drop. Although the triceps reflex is present, altered sensation is noted over the region of the anatomical snuffbox on the affected side.

8. Perioperative care: Critical care

A. Anaphylactic shock
B. Cardiogenic-septic shock with inappropriate heart rate
C. Cardiogenic shock: inflow obstruction
D. Cardiogenic shock: outflow obstruction
E. Cardiogenic shock: pump failure
F. Hypovolaemic shock: fluid redistribution
G. Hypovolaemic shock: fluid loss
H. Neurogenic shock
I. Septic shock

For each of the following situations, select the single most likely diagnosis from the options listed. Each option may be used once, more than once, or not at all.

1. A 72-year-old female undergoes a laparotomy for small bowel obstruction. Her comorbidities include diabetes, two previous myocardial infarctions, a permanent cardiac pacemaker and a 40-pack-year smoking history. Intraoperatively, a small amount of faecal contamination is noted but after a thorough peritoneal washout, the patient remains stable in the immediately postoperative period. Five hours after surgery, she becomes hypotensive with a blood pressure of 84/50 mmHg, heart rate of 70/min and temperature of 37°C.

2. A 45-year-old female is admitted to hospital for chemotherapy for her endometrial cancer, which is known to have extensive pelvic spread on CT imaging. Following her chemotherapy, she initially becomes hypoxic, and subsequently hypotensive with a blood pressure of 80/40 mmHg, heart rate of 140/min, temperature of 37°C and oxygen saturation of 79% on room air. Her ECG confirms sinus tachycardia and her serum haemoglobin level is 11.5 g/dL.

3. A 20-year-old painter presents to the Emergency Department after falling from scaffolding 2.8 m in height. The primary and secondary survey suggested a T2 vertebral fracture with complete neurological deficit below this point. While the patient is in the Radiology department, his blood pressure falls to 80/36 mmHg, and his heart rate drops to 45/min. His oxygen saturations fall to 85% on room air, while he becomes increasingly confused.

9. Professional behaviour and leadership: Patient safety

A. 0%

B. 0.2–0.5%

C. 1–2%

D. 4–5%

E. 10–12%

F. 20–25%

G. 40–50%

H. 60–80%

I. Over 80%

For each of the following situations, select the single most likely risk of complications from the options listed. Each option may be used only once.

1. A 53-year-old male with no previous medical history is found to have a 6.6 cm abdominal aortic aneurysm (AAA) as part of a national AAA screening programme. He is scheduled to undergo an open AAA repair. What is his risk of mortality from the procedure?

2. A 55-year-old female singer undergoes an elective thyroid lobectomy for early thyroid follicular adenocarcinoma. What is her risk of developing hoarseness of voice from her procedure?

3. A 46-year-old female undergoes an elective laparoscopic cholecystectomy for a 3-month history of symptomatic cholelithiasis. What is her risk of sustaining an injury to the common bile duct during this procedure?

10. The assessment and management of the surgical patient: Planning investigations

A. Barium swallow
B. Bronchoscopy
C. Computed tomography
D. Endoscopic ultrasonography
E. Colonoscopy
F. Endoscopic retrograde cholangiopancreatography
G. Laparoscopy
H. Magnetic resonance cholangiopancreatography
I. Magnetic resonance imaging

For each of the following situations, select the single most appropriate investigation from the options listed. Each option may be used once, more than once, or not at all.

1. A 32-year-old woman is seen in the pre-assessment clinic in preparation for a laparoscopic cholecystectomy. She describes a recent history of severe, right upper quadrant pain and vomiting. On direct questioning, she admits to passing dark urine and pale, oily stools. She is visibly jaundiced on examination. Blood tests reveal a bilirubin level of 65 mg/dL and ALP of 240 IU/L. Abdominal ultrasonography shows multiple small, mobile stones within the gallbladder, and dilatation of the common bile duct, with a small stone within it.

2. A 54-year-old chronic smoker is referred by his GP for upper gastrointestinal endoscopy for a recent onset of dysphagia. At endoscopy, a malignant-looking stricture is visualized in the distal third of the oesophagus, from which multiple biopsies are taken. The surgeon then organizes an ultrasound scan of the liver and a subsequent PET-CT scan, which altogether exclude metastatic disease. Which of the listed investigations should be performed to assess the patient's suitability for surgery?

3. An anxious 78-year-old woman is referred to the upper gastrointestinal outpatient clinic with a 3-month history of vague upper abdominal discomfort, nausea and unintentional weight loss. She appears cachectic but her physical examination is otherwise unremarkable. An upper gastrointestinal endoscopy does not reveal any abnormality but an ultrasound scan of her abdomen reveals a dilated common bile duct in the absence of gallstones.

11. Perioperative care: Critical care

A. Continuous positive airway pressure ventilation
B. Extracorporeal membrane oxygenation
C. High-frequency jet insufflation
D. High-frequency positive pressure ventilation
E. Intermittent mandatory ventilation
F. Intermittent positive pressure ventilation
G. Positive end-expiratory pressure ventilation
H. Pressure-controlled continuous mandatory ventilation
I. Pressure-controlled intermittent mandatory ventilation
J. Pressure support ventilation

For each of the following situations, select the single most appropriate means of ventilation from the options listed. Each option may be used once, more than once, or not at all.

1. A 75-year-old man is undergoing an elective left hemicolectomy for colorectal malignancy. The consultant anaesthetist describes to the patient the method of ventilation that he will be subjected to following the induction of general anaesthesia.

2. A 69-year-old man is admitted to the Intensive Care Unit following the emergency endovascular repair of a ruptured abdominal aortic aneurysm. The consultant intensive care physician subsequently observes that the patient's physiological parameters have stabilized and decides to wean the patient off the ventilator using a specific mode of ventilation.

3. A 30-year-old cyclist is brought to the Emergency Department following a road traffic accident. The initial clinical assessment and diagnostic imaging suggest extensive haemorrhage into the thoracic and abdominal cavities, necessitating a right thoracotomy and laparotomy. Although haemostasis is eventually achieved, the patient develops a systemic inflammatory response syndrome following a 15-unit blood transfusion. It is noted that despite aggressive attempts at ventilation, the patient's partial pressure of oxygen (PaO_2) demonstrates a steady drop. At this point, the consultant intensive care physician considers the most appropriate form of ventilation for the patient.

12. Professional behaviour and leadership: Clinical governance

A. Clinical audit
B. Complaints and patient advice liaison
C. Education and training
D. Multidisciplinary team approach
E. Patient and public involvement
F. Clinical effectiveness and research
G. Risk management
H. Staffing and management
I. Using information and information technology

For each of the following situations, select the most accurately represented pillar of clinical governance from the options listed. Each option may be used once, more than once, or not at all.

1. A junior doctor retrospectively collects data regarding the preoperative investigations performed on all elective surgical patients, to assess local compliance with NICE guidelines on preoperative assessment.

2. A surgical registrar submits a critical incident report for a patient who has been admitted to the surgical ward from the Emergency Department without having been formally assessed and accepted for admission by the surgical team.

3. A surgical trainee undergoes an appraisal with her educational supervisor, which involves identifying areas of weakness and opportunities for personal development.

13. The assessment and management of the surgical patient: Appropriate prescribing

A. Amoxicillin
B. Augmentin
C. Ciprofloxacin
D. Clindamycin
E. Gentamicin
F. Imipenem
G. Meropenem
H. Metronidazole
I. Penicillin V
J. Tazocin
K. Teicoplanin

For each of the following situations, select the single most appropriate antibiotic therapy from the options listed. Each option may be used once, more than once, or not at all.

1. A 45-year-old male is admitted to the Intensive Care Unit for severe alcohol-induced pancreatitis, associated with over 30% pancreatic necrosis, as suggested by abdominal CT imaging. The patient undergoes a CT-guided needle aspiration and culture of the necrotic tissue, which confirms the presence of infective necrosis.

2. A 25-year-old male undergoes an emergency splenectomy for traumatic rupture of his spleen following a road traffic accident. In the immediate postoperative period, he is commenced on lifelong antibiotic prophylaxis. The patient has no known drug allergies.

3. An 84-year-old nursing home resident presents to the Emergency Department with a 3-day history of worsening confusion and intermittent fever, which is deemed to be secondary to urosepsis. A culture performed on a urine sample from his long-term suprapubic catheter eventually grows extended-spectrum beta-lactamase producing organisms.

14. Perioperative care: Perioperative management of diabetes

A. Avoid oral anti-diabetic medication for 24 hours preoperatively, start on glucose-potassium-insulin (GKI) infusion, and restart oral anti-diabetic medication with first postoperative meal

B. Avoid oral anti-diabetic medication on the morning of surgery, avoid GKI infusion, and restart only gliclazide postoperatively

C. Avoid oral anti-diabetic medication on the morning of surgery, avoid GKI infusion, and restart oral anti-diabetic medication with first postoperative meal

D. Have breakfast and subcutaneous (SC) insulin 6 hours prior to surgery, and continue clear fluids until 2 hours preoperatively; keep starved thereafter, with hourly blood glucose monitoring

E. Have breakfast and SC insulin 6 hours prior to surgery; keep starved thereafter, with hourly blood glucose monitoring

F. Continue usual SC insulin regimen, monitor blood glucose and start on GKI infusion on the morning of surgery; restart usual SC insulin regimen after normal feeding pattern is re-established

G. Continue usual SC insulin regimen, monitor blood glucose and start on GKI infusion on the morning of surgery; restart usual SC insulin regimen with first meal

H. Keep starved from midnight and commence GKI infusion on the morning of surgery

I. Stop SC insulin and start GKI infusion 24 hours preoperatively; restart usual SC insulin regimen with first meal

For each of the following perioperative scenarios, select the single most appropriate regimen for diabetic control from the options listed. Each option may be used once, more than once, or not at all.

1. A 55-year-old diabetic man, who takes metformin and gliclazide, presents to the Emergency Department with severe renal colic. He subsequently undergoes an intravenous pyelogram and retrograde ureteric stenting. On the following morning, his serum biochemistry reveals that his estimated glomerular filtration rate is 22 mL/min/1.73m^2 and his blood glucose level is 10 mmol/L.

2. A 65-year-old insulin-dependent diabetic patient is kept starved from midnight for an elective right hemicolectomy. She is usually on a multiple-injection regimen of long-acting Lantus® insulin.

3. A 6-year-old diabetic boy is listed first on the afternoon operating list for an elective circumcision. His blood glucose level, which is usually well controlled, is measure to be 9 mmol/L on admission.

15. The assessment and management of the surgical patient: Case work-up and evaluation

A. T1N1M0
B. T1N2M0
C. T2N1M0
D. T2N2M0
E. T3N1M0
F. T3N2M0
G. T3N3M0
H. T4N1M0
I. T4N2M0
J. T4N3M0

For each of the following situations, select the single most likely TNM (tumour, node, metastasis) stage from the options listed. Each option may be used once, more than once, or not at all.

1. A 65-year-old man undergoes a radical nephrectomy for localized renal cell carcinoma. The histopathology report of the resected specimen describes a tumour of 9 cm diameter that is confined to the kidney, with two out of eight nodes positive.

2. A 40-year-old man undergoes an excision biopsy of a malignant melanoma in his right foot, which measures 3 mm in diameter, together with radical lymph node dissection in his right groin. The histopathology report confirms a malignant melanoma with two out of ten nodes positive.

3. A 30-year-old woman is referred to the breast clinic for a suspicious right-sided breast lump. Examination reveals a hard, mobile lump that is 3 cm in diameter and in the upper outer quadrant of her right breast, with no overlying skin changes. The patient is also found to have palpable, mobile lymph nodes in her right axilla. No other lymphadenopathy is evident on examination, and fine-needle aspiration cytology of the lump subsequently confirms breast cancer.

16. Perioperative care: Critical care

A. Bladder scan, flush catheter and replace catheter if necessary
B. Insert urinary catheter, check renal function and administer intravenous fluid therapy, guided by urine output
C. Perform cystoscopy and insert a retrograde double J ureteric stent
D. Administer fluid challenge with 250 mL of colloid
E. Commence haemodialysis
F. Commence haemofiltration
G. Administer inotropic support and furosemide infusion
H. Measure intra-abdominal pressure via urinary catheter
I. Perform percutaneous nephrostomy
J. Administer renal-dose dopamine

For each of the following situations, select the single most appropriate therapeutic option listed. Each option may be used once, more than once, or not at all.

1. A 68-year-old male presents to the Emergency Department with a 3-month history of anorexia, lethargy and lower urinary tract symptoms, such as hesitancy, poor stream and intermittent dribbling. Examination reveals a dehydrated patient with moderate suprapubic discomfort and bladder distension to the level of the umbilicus. Digital rectal examination confirms a significantly enlarged but benign-feeling prostate. A bladder scan suggests a residual volume of 1.8 litres, and renal function tests reveal a serum urea level of 34 mmol/L and a serum creatinine level of 450 µmol/L.

2. A 43-year-old female undergoes an exploratory laparotomy for penetrating abdominal trauma. During the procedure, she is found to have sustained a minor liver laceration, from which any haemorrhage is controlled. In the early postoperative period, she develops a distended and tender abdomen. Her urine output is found to drop steadily and she becomes progressively more acidotic, with an elevated serum lactate.

3. A 55-year-old female presents with a 2-day history of fever, dysuria and right-sided loin pain. She is found to be septic with a temperature of 39°C, heart rate of 120/min and blood pressure of 102/75 mmHg. Renal function tests reveals acute renal failure, while renal ultrasound imaging reveals right-sided hydronephrosis and proximal hydroureter. A CT urogram subsequently confirms an obstruction in the middle third of the right ureter, without any obvious cause identified.

17. The assessment and management of the surgical patient: Clinical decision-making

A. Angioplasty
B. Aorto-bifemoral bypass
C. Axillobifemoral bypass
D. Embolectomy
E. Femoro-distal bypass
F. Femoro-femoral bypass
G. Femoro-popliteal bypass
H. Lumbar sympathectomy
I. Profundoplasty

For each of the following situations, select the single most appropriate management option listed. Each option may be used once, more than once, or not at all.

1. A 68-year-old retired brewer is referred by his GP to the vascular surgeons for a 6-month history of progressively worsening right buttock and thigh claudication. His current claudication distance is 100 metres on flat ground and he is asymptomatic on the contralateral side. The patient mentions that he quit smoking two months prior to presentation. Examination reveals a full complement of pulses in the left lower limb but no pulses on the right side. An arterial duplex scan and angiography reveal a 12 cm occlusion of the right common and external iliac arteries. No other abnormalities are demonstrated.

2. A 77-year-old pub manager is referred by his GP to the vascular surgeons for a 2-month history of bilateral leg pain at rest. He has a significant history of peripheral vascular disease, including bilateral femoro-popliteal bypasses, and admits to continual heavy smoking. Examination reveals no palpable pulses in either leg, and subsequent vascular imaging demonstrates occlusion of both femoro-popliteal bypass grafts. The extent of occlusion precludes any further angioplasty, stenting or arterial reconstruction.

3. A 70-year-old woman presents to her GP with a 6-week history of progressively worsening, bilateral buttock pain. Her claudication distance is 100 metres on flat ground but she usually stops before achieving this distance due to breathlessness. Her past medical history includes stable angina and a myocardial infarction seven years previously. Subsequent vascular imaging reveals a severely stenosed aorta with multiple stenoses of both iliac arteries. Both femoral arteries are found to be patent with good run-off below the knees.

18. **Assessment and management of patients with trauma (including the multiply injured patient): Investigation and management**

    A. Admit for 24-hour observation
    B. Burr hole drainage
    C. Craniotomy and evacuation of haematoma
    D. Craniotomy and insertion of intracranial pressure monitoring device
    E. Computed tomography scan of head
    F. Discharge from hospital
    G. Intubation and ventilation
    H. Magnetic resonance imaging scan of head
    I. Plain radiography of skull

    For each of the following situations, select the single most appropriate investigative or management option listed. Each option may be used once, more than once, or not at all.

    1. A 27-year-old intoxicated male is brought to the Emergency Department by ambulance, after having been assaulted on his face with a baseball bat. On initial assessment, his eyes open spontaneously and he is able to follow commands, but makes incomprehensible sounds and appears generally uncomfortable. A CT scan of his head reveals bilateral mandibular fractures.

    2. A 45-year-old cricket player is struck on his left temporal region by a cricket ball. His teammates claim that he collapsed and subsequently remained unconscious for ten minutes. Two hours following his injury, in the Emergency Department, he becomes drowsy and develops right-sided weakness and contralateral pupillary dilatation. An urgent CT scan of his head reveals a left-sided, biconvex, high-attenuation lesion overlying the temporoparietal cortices.

    3. A 75-year-old female presents to the Emergency Department approximately 36 hours after sustaining a head injury from a mechanical fall. Her husband is concerned that she has become confused, drowsy and unsteady on her feet. A CT scan of her head confirms a low-density crescentic lesion overlying the left parietal cortex.

19. The assessment and management of the surgical patient: Investigations and management

A. Anti-androgen therapy

B. CT urography

C. Flexible cystoscopy

D. Cystoscopy and retrograde ureteric stent insertion

E. Intravenous urography

F. Percutaneous nephrostomy formation

G. Retrograde urethrography

H. Suprapubic catheterization

I. Three-way urethral catheterization and bladder irrigation

J. Transrectal ultrasonography and biopsy

K. Two-way urethral catheterization

For each of the following situations, select the single most appropriate immediate investigation or management option listed. Each option may be used once, more than once, or not at all.

1. A 27-year-old biker is involved in a high-speed collision with another motorcycle. Despite being thrown nine metres from his vehicle, he appears well on arrival to the Emergency Department. The primary and secondary surveys are normal, apart from fresh blood noted at the patient's external urethral meatus.

2. An 84-year-old gentleman presents to the Emergency Department with a 24-hour history of suprapubic pain and oliguria. He has no significant past medical history. Abdominal examination reveals a tender, enlarged bladder; and digital rectal examination reveals an asymmetrically enlarged, hard and nodular prostate gland. A urethral catheter is inserted but drains only 10 mL per hour of urine. Serum biochemistry reveals the following: Na 136 mmol/L, K 5.9 mmol/L, urea 63 mmol/L and creatinine 520 µmol/L. An urgent ultrasound of the urinary tract demonstrates bilateral hydronephrosis and hydroureter.

3. A 46-year-old policeman presents to the Emergency Department with a 4-hour history of excruciating, colicky, right-sided abdominal pain radiating from his loin to his groin. He had undergone a left nephrectomy for penetrating renal trauma 3 years previously. He is apyrexial and haemodynamically stable on examination, although he finds it difficult to keep still due to the pain. Plain radiography and subsequent non-contrast CT imaging confirm the presence of a 5 mm opacity in the right ureter, at the level of the L4 vertebra. Serum biochemistry reveals the following: Na 136 mmol/L, K 5.4 mmol/L, urea 21.5 mmol/L and creatinine 430 µmol /L.

4. A 92-year-old gentleman is referred urgently to the Emergency Department by his GP for a 48-hour history of painless macroscopic haematuria with clots. Over the last 12 hours, he has found it increasingly difficult to pass urine, and is now in considerable discomfort. Examination reveals an enlarged bladder and moderate suprapubic tenderness. A digital rectal examination is unremarkable.

20. Surgical care of the paediatric patient: History, examination, and assessment of neonates and children

A. Volvulus neonatorum

B. Hirschsprung's disease

C. Infantile hypertrophic pyloric stenosis

D. Necrotizing enterocolitis

E. Meconium ileus

F. Duodenal atresia

G. Anorectal atresia

H. Tracheoesophageal fistula

I. Intussusception

For each of the following situations, select the single most likely diagnosis from the options listed. Each option may be used once, more than once, or not at all.

1. A 6-week-old male infant is brought to the Emergency Department with a 3-day history of vomiting and reluctance to feed. The infant's vomitus contains partly digested food (i.e. milk) but no evidence of bile. The child appears dehydrated, and abdominal examination reveals a lump under the right costal margin when the child is given a 'test feed'.

2. A 5-day-old baby boy is brought to the Emergency Department by anxious parents who state that the baby has persistently been vomiting bilious fluid, and is unable to feed. Examination reveals a soft abdomen with no palpable masses. The child has not opened his bowels since passing the first meconium stool.

3. A 6-week-old baby boy is brought to the Emergency Department with a history of recurrent respiratory tract infections and intermittent vomiting. The parents describe that the baby appears blue and chokes whenever he is fed. They are concerned that although these symptoms have been present since birth, they are now considerably worsening. Physical examination of the child is unremarkable.

21. **The assessment and management of the surgical patient: Clinical decision-making**

   A. Anal cancer
   B. Breast cancer
   C. Colorectal cancer
   D. Ewing's sarcoma
   E. Leukaemia
   F. Non-small cell lung cancer
   G. Oesophageal cancer
   H. Small cell lung caner
   I. Testicular teratoma

   For each of the following descriptions, select the single most likely indication for chemotherapy from the options listed. Each option may be used once, more than once, or not at all.

   1. This chemosensitive tumour may be managed with curative intent using platinum-containing combination chemotherapy.

   2. Chemotherapy containing 5-fluorouracil (5-FU) may increase the disease-free survival interval in 10–12% of patients following surgical resection of this type of malignancy, although it cannot be used with curative intent in patients with metastatic disease.

   3. This tumour is highly chemosensitive and has a response rate of 80% to palliative chemotherapy, even in advanced disease. Chemotherapy has been shown to extend the median survival of affected patients from 3 months to 18 months.

22. Basic surgical skills: Incisions

A. Bilateral anterolateral thoracotomy ('clamshell')
B. Left anterolateral thoracotomy
C. Left posterolateral thoracotomy
D. Median sternotomy
E. Right anterolateral thoracotomy
F. Right posterolateral thoracotomy
G. Right vertical infra-axillary incision
H. Transsternal anterior thoracotomy

For each of the following situations, select the single most appropriate means of accessing the thoracic cavity from the options listed. Each option may be used once, more than once, or not at all.

1. A 65-year-old man attends the preoperative assessment clinic after being diagnosed with localized, primary squamous cell bronchogenic carcinoma of the right middle lobe. He is keen to undergo surgery but wonders where the scar from the operation is likely to be.

2. A 25-year-old motorcyclist is brought to the Emergency Department after colliding into a glass window, and sustaining penetrating trauma to the right side of his neck. Chest radiography reveals a complete opacification of the right lung field. Upon chest drain insertion, 1600 mL of fresh blood is immediately drained. The physician in charge decides to perform an emergency thoracotomy.

3. A 55-year-old man consults his GP for progressively worsening, symptomatic mitral valve disease. He is eventually referred to a cardiothoracic surgeon, who, prior to preoperative workup, explains the most likely operative procedure for the mitral valve replacement.

23. Professional behaviour and leadership: Medical statistics

A. Kaplan–Meier
B. Logrank test
C. Multiple regression
D. Negative predictive value
E. Positive predictive value
F. Receiver operating characteristic (ROC)
G. Sensitivity
H. Simple regression
I. Specificity
J. Type I
K. Type II

For each of the following descriptions, select the single most accurate statistical test or concept from the options listed. Each option may be used once, more than once, or not at all.

1. An academic surgeon wishes to perform a meta-analysis of studies to assess the survival outcome after endovascular aneurysm repair for ruptured abdominal aortic aneurysms. She wishes to use a specific diagram to express her survival data for this purpose.

2. A consultant surgeon wishes to teach his medical students about certain cancer screening programmes in the UK. He describes a particular term that indicates the proportion of patients with normal screening test results who are truly free from disease.

3. An academic surgeon becomes unsure about the validity of results and conclusions from his study after he learns that the true null hypothesis had been incorrectly rejected due to statistical oversight. Which of the above terms best describes the error made in the study?

24. Basic surgical skills: Principles of diathermy

A. Burns
B. Capacitance coupling
C. Channelling
D. Conduction
E. Collateral thermal damage
F. Disruption of active electrode
G. Explosion
H. Poor heat distribution
I. Surgical smoke toxicity

For each of the following situations, select the single most specific description of the mechanism of diathermy-induced injury from the options listed. Each option may be used once, more than once, or not at all.

1. An unexpected ignition occurs when the surgeon employs the use of diathermy on the large bowel during an emergency Hartmann's procedure.

2. The use of monopolar diathermy to subcutaneous fat within an upper midline incision induces a transient arrhythmia in a patient with a cardiac pacemaker.

3. Inadvertent injury to the liver is caused by the accidental use of metal laparoscopic ports together with plastic insulator cuffs during a laparoscopic cholecystectomy.

4. Failed attempts at haemostasis during a paediatric circumcision in a child with haemophilia lead to the use of diathermy, which inadvertently causes coagulation damage to the child's penis.

1. Answers: 1-J; 2-D; 3-C; 4-G

1. The history and symptoms in this patient are suggestive of dermatofibroma, which is also known as fibrous histiocytoma or sclerosing haemangioma. Dermatofibromas are firm ('woody'), well-defined, indolent, and single or multiple freely mobile nodules usually found over the extremities. They are usually observed in young or middle-aged patients, and are more common in women. Mild trauma or insect bites may trigger their incidence, leading to the suggestion that these lesions are not true tumours, but instead, the result of a tissue reaction. Whilst some tumours are histologically cellular in nature (i.e. being composed largely of histiocytes), others are fibrous (i.e. being composed of fibroblasts and collagen); others feature a predominantly angiomatous component. The management of dermatofibromas is by simple excision.

2. The signs and symptoms of this patient are suggestive of lupus vulgaris (i.e. tuberculosis of the skin). This condition usually occurs in individuals between the ages of 10–25 years. The lesions appear as single or multiple 'apple jelly-like' cutaneous nodules, commonly over the face and neck. They tend to heal in one area as the disease process extends to another. The mucous membrane of the mouth and nose are sometimes affected, either primarily, or as an extension of disease from the face. Infection of the nasal cavity may lead to the necrosis of the underlying cartilage. Oedema occurs if the fibrosis induced by the disease obstructs the normal lymphatic drainage. The management of lupus vulgaris is primarily by anti-tubercular chemotherapy.

3. This patient presents with the classical signs of an infected sebaceous cyst (i.e. epidermoid cyst). Sebaceous cysts are intradermal lesions containing keratin and its breakdown products, surrounded by a wall of stratified squamous keratinizing epithelium. They commonly occur over the face, chest, and shoulders, and may be inherited in an autosomal dominant fashion. Sebaceous cysts feature a characteristic punctum, usually in the centre of the lesion, which blocks the sebaceous outflow. Treatment is by surgical excision, during which the complete removal of the cyst wall is essential in minimizing recurrence.

4. The signs and symptoms of this patient are suggestive of seborrhoeic keratosis (i.e. basal cell papilloma or seborrhoeic wart). Seborrhoeic keratoses are benign tumours caused by the overgrowth of epidermal keratinocytes. The disease commonly occurs in individuals who are over 40 years of age. The lesions are frequently pigmented and often develop as single or multiple entities that are round or oval-shaped, slightly greasy lesions with a 'stuck on' appearance. Sometimes they occur in crops in sun-exposed areas (e.g. the trunk, face and arms) and are often characterized by a network of crypts. Multiple seborrhoeic keratoses may be associated with an internal malignancy (Leser–Trélat sign).

2. Answers: 1-H; 2-F; 3-D

1. This patient's age and presenting history support a diagnosis of inflammatory bowel disease. In an elderly patient, the finding of left iliac fossa tenderness would be more suggestive of

diverticulitis. In addition, the symptoms of blood and mucus per rectum are more in keeping with ulcerative colitis than Crohn's disease. The diagnosis is confirmed by sigmoidoscopy and biopsy, which will reveal a friable granular mucosa with an inflammatory infiltrate, goblet cell depletion, glandular distortion, mucosal ulcers and crypt abscesses. This is in contrast to Crohn's disease, which involves the characteristic transmural granulomatous inflammation, predisposing to stricturing, with evidence of skip lesions (i.e. giving a 'cobblestone' appearance on endoscopy).

2. This patient is most likely to have undergone surgery for uterine malignancy, together with adjuvant radiotherapy. Her symptoms are typical of acute radiation enteritis, which may feature non-specific abdominal discomfort, bloody diarrhoea, tenesmus, and features of gastrointestinal obstruction, malabsorption and proctitis. Radiation enteritis is caused by radiation doses exceeding 50 Gy (usually to the pelvis); the ileum and rectum are most commonly affected. Acute radiation enteritis occurs at the time of exposure and usually persists for 6 weeks; it occurs in approximately 50% of patients undergoing abdominopelvic radiotherapy. Chronic radiation enteritis is diagnosed if symptoms persist for more than 3 months. Although the treatment of radiation enteritis is largely symptomatic, radiation proctitis may respond well to local steroid therapy. Surgery may be considered in life-threatening situations, such as obstruction or perforation.

3. Whipple's operation is a radical procedure that aims to cure pancreatic carcinoma or cholangiocarcinoma (i.e. where lesions are extrahepatic and periampullary), or, occasionally, chronic pancreatitis. It involves resecting most of the extrahepatic biliary system, the entire duodenum, the distal stomach and the head of the pancreas. Anastomoses are formed between the remaining structures (e.g. the tail of the pancreas to the jejunal stump; and the bile duct to the side of the jejunum). This scenario involves a pylorus-preserving pancreaticodudenectomy, which is a modified Whipple's procedure that preserves the pylorus. The nature of this operation requires the patient to remain nil-by-mouth for a prolonged postoperative period, during which time nutritional support is administered via a feeding jejunostomy (or by total parenteral nutrition). A trial of enteral feeding is therefore the likely cause of diarrhoea in this patient. As the patient is likely to have received intravenous antibiotics, pseudomembranous colitis should also form part of the differential diagnosis of his diarrhoea.

3. Answers: 1-I; 2-G; 3-A

1. Acute pyelonephritis is an acute infection of the renal parenchyma, which frequently involves an ascending infection from the urinary bladder. The common clinical features include dysuria, loin pain, pyrexia, rigors, and flu-like symptoms. The combination of these features with a urine dipstick result indicative of infection, should prompt the rapid commencement of empirical antibiotic therapy (e.g. with broad-spectrum cephalosporin or a quinolone) until the urine culture results are known. Treatment should continue for 14 days, and for longer in cases of complicated pyelonephritis. The patient should also receive bed rest until systemic symptoms and local tenderness resolve, analgesia, and an increased fluid intake (e.g. 3 litres daily). It is vital for surgeons to remember that pyelonephritis in the presence of urinary tract obstruction is a urological emergency, which must be diagnosed and managed rapidly (e.g. with percutaneous nephrostomy) to avoid the rapid progression to septic shock. Open surgery is only required if a complication such as a perinephric abscess develops, in which case, the abscess is drained via a loin incision.

2. This patient has developed pneumonia whilst undergoing invasive ventilation on the Intensive Care Unit. Acinetobacter baumannii is a prevalent nosocomial pathogen, especially in patients who undergo mechanical ventilation. It is also known as an opportunistic pathogen that may cause significant sepsis in elderly or immunocompromised patients. The resultant infection

is challenging to treat and is associated with a high mortality rate, largely due to the patients' existing poor premorbid status. Imipenem is the first-line antibiotic therapy for A. *baumannii* strains that are sensitive to it, along with strict infection control measures. Other treatment options include tigecycline and aminoglycosides.

3. Breast abscesses are commonly associated with lactation but may also occur in non-lactating women, and as a consequence of localised skin infection. In lactating women, the causative organism is most commonly *Staphylococcus aureus* but in non-lactating women, causative pathogens include *Streptococci* and anaerobes. The treatment of choice for *S. aureus* infection is penicillin, with the first-line therapy most commonly being a penicillinase-resistant β-lactam antibiotic, such as flucloxacillin. Patients who are penicillin-resistant may receive erythromycin. Rare organisms causing breast abscesses include *Mycobacterium tuberculosis* and *Actinomyces spp.* In non-lactating women, the main differential diagnosis is inflammatory breast cancer, which must be clinically excluded. Other causes or predisposing factors (e.g. diabetes mellitus) for the breast abscess must also be carefully excluded. Breast milk should be obtained for culture and sensitivity, if possible. Improvements to the breast feeding technique and the infant's attachment to the mother's breast should be suggested, if necessary.

4. Answers: 1-C; 2-E; 3-D

The introduction to the question briefly mentions ARDS as the indication for ventilation in the three scenarios. The aim in these cases is to provide reasonable oxygenation and CO_2 removal without causing further damage to the lungs. This compromise is achieved by maintaining permissible hypercapnoea to CO_2 of 10–15 kPa without evidence of respiratory acidosis or cerebral oedema, and an acceptable level of hypoxaemia to PaO_2 of 8 kPa. This can be achieved by the aforementioned ventilation methods.

1. Continuous positive airway pressure ventilation (CPAP) involves the use of continuous positive pressure to maintain an uninterrupted level of positive airway pressure. CPAP is functionally similar to positive end-expiratory pressure ventilation (PEEP), although PEEP involves an applied pressure against exhalation, while CPAP is a pressure applied by a constant flow. As the ventilator does not cycle during this process, no additional pressure is provided above the level of CPAP, requiring patients to initiate their own breaths. CPAP tends to recruit alveoli and expand collapsed areas of lung, thereby increasing functional residual capacity and improving oxygenation. It is typically used for patients who have longstanding respiratory problems, such as sleep apnoea, although it may also be used for early ARDS, as in this scenario.

2. As conventional volume-controlled ventilation may induce barotrauma to healthy lungs, pressure-controlled ventilation (PCV) may be used in certain situations instead. PCV rapidly achieves a fixed pressure throughout the breath (i.e. creating a 'square pressure waveform') by delivering a decelerating inspiratory flow pattern. This results in a tidal volume that varies with lung compliance and resistance. PCV is closely monitored with alarms set for a minimal acceptable tidal volume (and/or minute volume). Apart from the reduced risk of barotrauma from PCV, its other advantages include improved gas exchange due to decelerating flow, more homogenous ventilation in cases of distribution disorders, and improved compensation for any leaks. A disadvantage of PCV is that if an increase in airway resistance (or reduction in lung compliance) occurs, the delivered tidal volume decreases, and hypoventilation results.

3. During normal respiration, the inspiratory to expiratory ratio is 1:2. Due to the short time in inspiration and decreased lung compliance experienced in ARDS, this often leads to high inflation pressures. This may be inhibited by prolonging the inspiration to expiration ratio by inverse ratio ventilation (IRV), which is a method of ventilating the lung such that some inspired

air is not allowed to be exhaled. This creates an intrinsic positive-end expiratory pressure, allowing for a constant inflation of the lungs, ensuring that they remain 'recruited'. The primary goal of IRV is to improve oxygenation by forcing inspiratory time to be greater than expiratory time, thereby increasing the mean airway pressure and potentially improving oxygenation. However, this process is largely unnatural and uncomfortable for the patient, requiring deep sedation and paralysis. It may also result in hypercapnoea and haemodynamic instability. Although IRV is suggested to improve oxygenation in ARDS, it has never been proven to improve key clinical outcomes (e.g. mortality, duration of mechanical ventilation, duration of intensive care), potentially due to the fact that IRV is not considered as a mode of ventilation early enough after ARDS has been diagnosed.

5. Answers: 1-C; 2-A; 3-F

1. This clinical presentation is most likely to represent an acute extradural haematoma. After the primary injury occurs, the patient may or may not experience a transient loss of consciousness, followed by a period of lucidity. This is followed by the rapidly deteriorating consciousness that is usually seen in younger patients. It occurs secondarily to disruption of meningeal arteries, commonly due to a skull fracture (e.g. of the pterion, which overlies the middle meningeal artery). Rapid expansion of the haematoma leads to rapid compression of the skull contents (i.e. in keeping with the Monro-Kellie doctrine), and a rapid reduction in consciousness after a period of lucidity. The diagnosis should always be confirmed on CT scan (or subsequent lumbar puncture, if CT imaging is initially negative). The optimal treatment involves craniotomy, evacuation of the haematoma, control of the bleeding point, and restoration of the skull vault anatomy.

2. This presentation is most likely to represent a basal skull fracture. Skull fractures may be fractures of the cranial vault or basal skull fractures. Cranial vault fractures may be linear, comminuted or depressed. Depressed fractures should be elevated if they are causing compression of the brain or will leave a significant cosmetic defect. In contrast, basal skull fractures may involve the anterior cranial fossa or the petrous temporal bone. Fractures of the anterior cranial fossa may be suggested by cerebrospinal fluid rhinorrhoea (i.e. due to damage to the cribriform plate, often requiring formal dural repair); bilateral periorbital haematoma ('racoon eyes'); and subconjunctival haemorrhage (i.e. where the posterior margin cannot be ascertained. Fractures of the petrous temporal bone may be suggested by bleeding from the external auditory meatus, cerebrospinal fluid otorrhoea (i.e. through a torn tympanic membrane—this usually entails a linear injury not requiring formal dural repair); and bruising over the mastoid process (Battle's sign), which may take up to 48 hours to develop. Due to the risk of infection from basal skull fractures, antibiotics are given prophylactically against meningitis for at least 7 days (or, in the presence of a cerebrospinal fluid leak, until 7 days after the leak has ceased).

3. This presentation is most likely to represent a subdural haematoma. This most commonly occurs due to rupture of the cortical bridging veins, which connect the cranial venous system to the large intradural venous sinuses, and lie relatively unprotected in the subdural space. The subdural space is then slowly enlarged with extravasated blood, enlarging over time to cause a mass effect, resulting in raised intracranial pressure. Subdural haematomas are commonly observed in elderly patients days after a minor head injury, which patients may not even recall. They are bilateral in 30% of cases. Risk factors include cerebral atrophy, anticoagulation (which this patient is likely to be on for his atrial fibrillation) and coagulation disorders, other conditions that predispose to minor head injuries, (e.g. epilepsy or cardiovascular disease), and arachnoid cysts (seen in younger patients). After the diagnosis is confirmed on CT imaging, conservative management (i.e. steroid therapy over several weeks) may be undertaken in fully conscious adults. In adults with depressed conscious levels, the haematoma may be evacuated with 2-3 burr holes, following

saline irrigation and nursing in the 'head down' position (i.e. to prevent recollection). In infants, repeated needle aspiration through the anterior fontanelle may be used for haematoma evacuation; or subdural peritoneal shunting may be used for persistent subdural collections.

6. Answers: 1-B; 2-A; 3-G

1. This child has developed erysipelas, which is a rapidly spreading streptococcal infection of the skin and subcutaneous tissue, characterized by cellulitis and lymphangitis. It is almost inevitably due to infection by *Streptococcus pyogenes*, but occasionally, other beta-haemolytic *Streptococci*, or rarely, *Staphylococci*, may be responsible. The disease is commonly seen in infants, children and the elderly. The development of erysipelas commonly involves bacterial inoculation in area any of skin trauma. Facial erysipelas is usually preceded by a streptococcal throat infection, suggesting that the patient's nasopharynx would be the source of infections in such instances. In addition, all the signs of inflammation with local lymphangitis and regional lymphadenopathy are present. Treatment involves symptomatic relief (i.e. bed rest with the head of the bed elevated; NSAIDS for pain and fever), and systemic antibiotic therapy.

2. This patient presents with signs and symptoms of a periareolar non-lactating breast infection. This involves the infection of non-dilated subareolar breast ducts, and most commonly affects young women, with a mean age of 32 years. The condition may present with periareolar inflammation and generalized breast tenderness, with or without nipple discharge. Examination may reveal nipple retraction, together with an associated inflammatory mass or abscess. Periductal mastitis is histologically characterized by active inflammation around non-dilated subareolar mammary ducts — in contrast to mammary duct ectasia, which commonly affects older women, the duct dilatation of periductal mastitis is less pronounced. The majority (90%) of women with periductal mastitis are smokers, therefore suggesting that smoking induces damage to the subareolar ducts, which then become infected with aerobic or anaerobic organisms (i.e. commonly *Staphylococcus aureus*, and occasionally *Enterococci*, anaerobic *Streptococci* and *Bacteroides* species). It must be remembered that in non-lactating women, the main differential diagnosis of such a presentation is inflammatory breast cancer, which must be excluded during clinical assessment.

3. Pseudomembranous colitis is a severe form of antibiotic-related colitis or diarrhoea. It is usually results from the toxin of *Clostridium difficile*, a Gram-positive, spore-forming aerobic bacillus. This commonly follows an antibiotic-induced change (e.g. from lincomycin, clindamycin, ampicillin, amoxicillin and cephalosporins) in the balance of normal gut flora, encouraging the overgrowth of *C. difficile*. In surgical patients, the condition frequently presents in the postoperative period, with worsening and eventually prostrating diarrhoea. This may develop into toxic megacolon, and may be fatal, especially in elderly patients. The condition is also associated with a high recurrence rate. The diagnosis is made from eliciting a history of recent antibiotic usage, by demonstrating *C. difficile* toxin in the faeces (i.e. using cell-culture assay or immunoassay), or by sigmoidoscopy or proctoscopy, which demonstrates punctate, adherent, yellow-white plaques on an inflamed rectal mucosa. The management involves stopping the offending antibiotic, followed by the use of oral metronidazole or vancomycin (metronidazole is commonly used as the first-line treatment due to its cost-effectiveness).

7. Answers: 1-C; 2-H; 3-E

1 and 3. The radial nerve arises from the spinal nerve roots C5–T1, and provides vital innervation to the dorsal aspect of the arm and forearm. It supplies the triceps, brachioradialis, all the wrist and finger extensors, and extensor pollicis longus and brevis to the thumb. The sensory supply of the radial nerve includes the dorsum of the thumb and the first dorsal web space, and

the dorsum of the forearm. The clinical pattern of disability from radial nerve lesions depends largely on the level of injury: in very high lesions where the radial nerve may be compressed in the axilla (e.g. high-speed RTA or inappropriate use of crutches), there is complete paralysis of the triceps, paralysis of the extensors supplied by the radial nerve (i.e. resulting in wrist drop), and an absent triceps reflex. In such lesions, there is sensory loss over the dorsum of the forearm, the dorsum of the thumb and the first dorsal web space. In high lesions, such as fractures of the humerus (particularly mid-shaft fractures, where the radial nerve lies in the spiral grove), or due to prolonged tourniquet pressure, there is weakness of the radial extensors of the wrist and numbness over the anatomical snuffbox. Such patterns of injury are also seen in patients who fall asleep with their arm dangling over the back of a chair ('Saturday night palsy'). The action of triceps and the triceps reflex may be preserved if the lesion is below the spiral grove in the humerus.

2. The ulnar nerve, which arises from the spinal nerve roots C8 and T1, is an important motor nerve of the hand. Disruptions to the ulnar nerve at the level of the wrist (i.e. usually from trauma), is the commonest cause of low ulnar nerve lesions. The nerve may also be affected by pressure from a deep ganglion. Ulnar nerve lesions at the level of the wrist produce hypothenar wasting and clawing of the hand due to the unopposed action of the long flexors, as well as sensory loss over the little and ring fingers. Finger abduction and adduction are both impaired, due to weakness of the dorsal and palmar interossei respectively. Weakness of adductor pollicis may be elicited as Froment's sign (i.e. inadvertent flexion of the thumb – using flexor pollicis longus – when the patient is instructed to grip a flat object between their thumb and index finger).

8. Answers: 1-B; 2-D; 3-H

1. The faecal contamination encountered during this patient's laparotomy increases her risk of postoperative intra-abdominal sepsis. The resultant sepsis (i.e. systemic inflammatory response syndrome with an infective focus) has caused peripheral vasodilatation and a subsequent fall in peripheral vascular resistance. As the patient's heart rate is fixed by her cardiac pacemaker, she is unable to compensate for this drop in systemic blood pressure by increasing her heart rate, thereby increasing her cardiac output. Although her blood pressure may temporarily respond to dobutamine, it may be worth considering resetting her cardiac pacemaker to permit a higher heart rate.

2. The clinical signs of acute hypoxia prior to developing hypovolaemia, suggest a cardiorespiratory cause for the patient's shock in this scenario. This is despite the patient's normal serum haemoglobin level, which alone is no indicator of normovolaemia, since haemoglobin levels tend not to fall drastically in the acute haemorrhagic state (i.e. as haemodilution takes time to occur). In consideration of this patient's diagnosis of endometrial cancer, extensive pelvic disease, and recent chemotherapy, the clinician must consider the diagnosis of cardiac outflow obstruction secondary to a large pulmonary embolus. Serum D-dimer may be measured as clinically indicated, and a CTPA should be performed to confirm or exclude the diagnosis.

3. Neurogenic shock is the most likely explanation for this young patient's clinical symptoms and signs, especially the combination of a high spinal lesion, hypotension and bradycardia. The neurogenic shock occurs as a result of disruption of both spinal cord and sympathetic tracts. The patient is hypotensive due to the loss of sympathetic vasomotor tone to the lower aspect of his body, and he is bradycardic due to the impairment of cardio-accelerator innervation. He is therefore hypotensive and unable to compensate for this by raising his heart rate. The initial management of this patient should be in accordance with the ATLS® guidelines, attending to the airway, breathing, and circulation first. After adequate fluid resuscitation, a combination of vasopressors and inotropes may be used to maintain haemodynamic stability.

9. Answers: 1-D; 2-C; 3-B

1. The current operative mortality rate from an elective open AAA repair is approximately 5%, and is approximately 2% for endovascular aneurysm repair (EVAR). Surgery should therefore be offered to those in whom the risk of rupture exceeds that of surgery; the estimated annual rupture rate of aneurysms larger than 6 cm is 10%, rising to over 30% for aneurysms larger than 8 cm. The 5-year survival of patients with aneurysms larger than 5 cm, who are not operated on, is approximately 20%. The UK Small Aneurysm Trial, a multicentre randomized control trial of early surgery versus surveillance of small AAA has revealed that elective repair of aneurysms smaller than 5.5 cm in diameter cannot be justified. It must be remembered that for emergency AAA repair, the operative mortality rises to 50%. Other common intraoperative risks associated with elective repair include haemorrhage and retroperitoneal haematoma, trash foot from distal emboli, graft occlusion, myocardial infarction and pneumonia.

2. The perioperative complications of thyroid surgery include recurrent laryngeal nerve damage (unilateral or bilateral), haemorrhage (causing tracheal compression and asphyxia), and damage to adjacent structures (e.g. trachea, oesophagus, laryngeal muscles). Bilateral recurrent laryngeal nerve damage presents as laryngeal obstruction after tracheal extubation, and requires emergency tracheostomy. Approximately 1–2% of patients develop such paralysis so preoperative laryngoscopy is vital to confirm premorbid vocal cord function. Early postoperative complications include local haemorrhage (now presenting as a rapid neck swelling, or significant blood in the drain), mediastinal haemorrhage (presenting as hypovolaemic shock), laryngeal oedema (inevitably causing voice hoarseness, and occasionally, acute airway obstruction), thyrotoxic crisis, and transient hypocalcaemia. Late complications include hypoparathyroidism (in 1% of patients), unilateral recurrent laryngeal nerve damage presenting as persistent hoarseness of voice (note that bilateral recurrent laryngeal nerve damage presents as laryngeal obstruction), and superior laryngeal nerve damage (presenting as a change in voice quality), and superior laryngeal nerve damage (presenting as a change in voice pitch). It is prudent to understand Semon's law, which states that in progressive recurrent laryngeal nerve palsy, the abductors are paralysed before the adductors (i.e. in incomplete paralysis, the cord will be brought to the midline by the adductors, but in complete paralysis it moves to the paramedian position.)

3. The risk of common bile duct injury during elective laparoscopic cholecystectomy is about 1 in 500. The majority of these injuries are noticed at the time of operation and repaired following conversion to an open procedure. It should be noted that the overall morbidity rate for the procedure varies between 1.6% and 11%, with the operative mortality being less than 0.08% to 0.7%. Apart from damage to the bile ducts, other complications of biliary surgery include retained stones in the biliary tree, biliary peritonitis secondary to bile leakage, haemorrhage (i.e. the cystic and hepatic arteries, and the liver bed, are all vulnerable to operative trauma and heavy bleeding), complications of pre-existing jaundice, ascending cholangitis, intraperitoneal abscesses in the gallbladder bed (or the peri-hepatic space), bowel injury, and other complications of surgery and anaesthesia (e.g. atelectasis, chest infection, wound infection, DVT, PE, etc.)

10. Answers: 1-F; 2-D; 3-C

1. The patient in this scenario manifests all of the signs, symptoms and investigative findings of obstructive jaundice. Urgent endoscopic retrograde cholangiopancreatography (ERCP) is warranted in such patients due to their high risk of developing cholangitis and pancreatitis from their existing cholestatic disesase. ERCP is of greater utility than magnetic resonance cholangiopancreatography (MRCP) in these instances due to the interventional capability of ERCP, which may be used to extract any obstructing stones, to perform a sphincterotomy, and to insert an

endoluminal biliary stent to facilitate bile drainage. It is vital that ERCP is performed prior to laparoscopic cholecystectomy, as a distal obstruction may result in an accumulation of back pressure, resulting in a 'blow out' of the cystic duct stump, predisposing to postoperative biliary peritonitis.

2. This patient demonstrates clear clinical, endoscopic and radiological evidence of non-metastatic distal oesophageal malignancy. Following the diagnosis of any oesophageal malignancy on endoscopy (and biopsy), a CT scan of the thorax and abdomen should be performed as part of locoregional staging and the preoperative assessment. The ultrasound scan of the liver, and PET-CT imaging, are useful adjuncts in detecting metastatic disease. In the absence of metastatic disease, endoscopic ultrasound is highly specific and highly sensitive in assessing the degree of local tumour invasion and operability. In oesophageal cancer involving the upper and middle thirds of the oesophagus, bronchoscopy may also be indicated to exclude bronchial involvement of the tumour.

3. The clinical findings of upper abdominal pain and weight loss, together with finding a dilated common bile duct in the absence of gallstones, should prompt the suspicion of carcinoma of the head of the pancreas (or a periampullary tumour) in this elderly patient. Computed tomography scanning provides excellent delineation of solid organs, and is therefore the investigation of choice to confirm or exclude hepatobiliary malignancy in this scenario. If this patient's abdominal ultrasound scan had revealed a dilated biliary tree in the presence of gallstones, MRCP may also be considered in the diagnostic work-up, due to its high sensitivity at interpreting soft tissue structures and biliary contrast.

11. Answers: 1-F; 2-I; 3-B

1. The administration of muscle relaxants (i.e. to facilitate abdominal surgery) during the induction of general anaesthesia will produce narcotic-induced apnoea, requiring the patient to undergo tracheal intubation and intermittent positive pressure ventilation (IPPV). During IPPV, which is a form of volume-controlled continuous mandatory ventilation, the ventilator provides a mechanical breath with either a pre-set tidal volume or peak pressure whenever the patient initiates a breath. The IPPV thereby allows for good relaxation with control of the patient's oxygenation, and elimination of carbon dioxide. It is useful to note that most ventilators feature a safety 'minimum ventilation rate' to avoid incidences of apnoea.

2. Pressure-controlled intermittent mandatory ventilation (formally known as 'synchronized intermittent mandatory ventilation' or SIMV) involves the ventilator delivering a pre-set pressure-limited mechanical breath at fixed intervals (e.g. of a few seconds). It is frequently employed as the method of weaning patients off mechanical ventilatory support. The transition from controlled mandatory ventilation to other modes that permit a patient's input into ventilation is not an exact science, but involves gradually decreasing the ventilation rate, thereby requiring the patient to take additional breaths beyond the ventilator-triggered breath. Continuous positive airway pressure (CPAP) ventilation and positive end-expiratory pressure (PEEP) ventilation are usually introduced as the patient gradually regains consciousness.

3. Extracorporeal membrane oxygenation (ECMO) is an extracorporeal technique of providing circulatory and respiratory support to patients who cannot independently maintain their cardiorespiratory function. Following the initial surgical cannulation, an ECMO specialist provides continuous monitoring for the duration of treatment. Common indications for ECMO include acute respiratory failure and cardiac failure (e.g. after major sepsis or trauma), and in neonates who need cardiorespiratory support. When applied to cadavers, ECMO can

also increase the viability of organs for transplant. The two most common methods of delivering ECMO are the veno-arterial and veno-venous methods. Despite its benefits, ECMO may cause neurological complications (e.g. subarachnoid haemorrhage, ischaemic watershed infarctions, hypoxic–ischaemic encephalopathy, unexplained coma, and brain death; as well as intraventricular haemorrhage in preterm infants), sepsis, bleeding (e.g. from heparin-induced thrombocytopenia), pulmonary haemorrhage/infarction, and aortic thrombosis.

12. Answers: 1-A; 2-G; 3-C

Clinical governance is a quality assurance process, which aims to ensure that certain standards of care are maintained and improved within the National Health Service (NHS), and that the NHS remains accountable to the general public. All the options listed, except for D and H, comprise the 7 pillars of clinical governance.

1. This scenario is an example of the audit process. Clinical audit is a review of current health practice against set standards, designed to ensure that clinicians provide the best level of care for their patients, and that they constantly seek to improve their practice where it is not measuring up to those standards. The audit cycle involves the following steps:

- Identifying an issue or problem through complaints or mistakes, or from national standards.
- Identifying standards to audit current practice against those drawn from the best available evidence.
- Collecting data on current practice for a specific group of patients during a pre-agreed period of clinical practice.
- Assessing the conformity of clinical practice with the standard. If the standard is not met, the reason for non-compliance should be identified so that it can be remedied.
- Implementing change: this process may include altering protocols, training staff, improving documentation, raising awareness, etc.
- Closing the loop and re-audit: after the changes have been implemented, re-audit should be performed after an agreed period of time to measure the impact of changes and to assess conformity to the previously defined standards.

2. Risk management entails having a robust system in place to understand, monitor and minimize risk to patients and staff, by learning from previous errors. It involves complying with protocols, learning from 'near misses' and consequential errors, reporting any significant adverse events by using formal critical incident reporting procedures, and promoting an open, 'blame-free' ethos to encourage the reporting of errors and shortfalls within the system. It is also vital to assess the chances of any risks identified, as well as their potential consequences, and thereafter, to implement processes to reduce the risk of such adverse events, as well as the severity of their consequences.

3. Continuing professional development (or 'continuing professional education') is the means by which doctors maintain their knowledge and skills related to their clinical practice. This often involves a structured approach to continual education to ensure competence to practice, and the progressive development of knowledge, skills and practical experience. The clinical governance pillar 'Education and training' emphasizes that adequate support be provided for clinicians, and other members of the multidisciplinary team, to remain competent in their various roles and to ensure that their skills are kept up-to-date. This may be achieved by attending courses and conferences, attending relevant examinations, undergoing regular work-based assessments, and by consistent peer-review and appraisals. This is consistent with the initiative of the General Medical Council to ensure that periodic revalidation is a vital and mandatory undertaking for all practising clinicians.

13. Answers: 1-F; 2-A; 3-G

1. The use of prophylactic antibiotics in patients with severe pancreatitis remains controversial, due to the risk of acquiring selective resistance by certain pathogenic species and fungal infections. Antibiotic therapy is generally reserved for patients who have been suggested to suffer from more than 30% pancreatic necrosis on CT imaging, in which case, prophylactic antibiotics may lead to a significant reduction in mortality. An aspirate of the necrotic tissue may be obtained and analysed for sensitivities, in order to guide antibiotic therapy. Imipenem has been found to be the most effective antibiotic therapy in this patient group. Patients should also be kept well hydrated and comfortable, and enteral feeding should be established as soon as patients are able to tolerate it.

2. Patients who have undergone a splenectomy are at an increased risk of developing overwhelming sepsis, particularly from encapsulated bacteria, such as *Pneumococci*, *Meningococci* and *Haemophilus influenzae*. Apart from ensuring that such patients are vaccinated against these organisms in the perioperative period, these patients should be prescribed lifelong antibiotic prophylaxis with amoxicillin (e.g. 250–500 mg/day; or erythromycin 250–500 mg/day for penicillin-allergic patients). Amoxicillin has the advantages of better absorption, having a broader spectrum, and having a longer shelf-life than penicillin. Finally, asplenic (or hyposplenic) patients should consider being vaccinated annually against the influenza virus.

3. Extended-spectrum beta-lactamase (ESBL) producing organisms include a spectrum of *Enterobacteriaceae*, *Klebsiella spp.* and *Escherichia coli*. These organisms produce beta-lactamase enzymes, which are highly effective in deactivating beta-lactam antibiotics. ESBL-producing organisms are generally multidrug resistant, and are largely resistant to quinolones and sulphonamides. The recent rise in the amount of third-generation cephalosporin usage has been implicated as a major cause for the proliferation of ESBL. The carbapenem class of antibiotics is commonly used to treat ESBL-related urosepsis, and since meropenem has been demonstrated to be the most effective carbapenem in-vitro, it is an acceptable choice of antibiotic therapy in this instance.

14. Answers: 1-B; 2-F; 3-D

1. Diabetic patients who take only oral anti-diabetic medication, who are undergoing minor surgery, should have all oral anti-diabetic medication omitted on the morning of surgery. Glucose-potassium-insulin (GKI) infusions should also be omitted in these patients if their blood glucose levels remain stable. Such oral anti-diabetic medication may be recommenced with the first postoperative meal, except for patients who are at a high risk of developing metformin-associated lactic acidosis, who should have their metformin omitted. An example of this would be the patient in this scenario, who has evidently developed postoperative renal impairment from the nephrotoxic contrast of the intravenous pyelogram.

2. For diabetic patients who are on subcutaneous (SC) regimens of insulin, insulin therapy should be maintained in the preoperative period, to reduce the risk of diabetic ketoacidosis if the GKI infusions are interrupted. Maintaining the SC insulin regimens in these patients also aids the smooth transition back onto SC insulin postoperatively. On the morning of surgery, blood glucose levels should be checked early, and the patient commenced on a GKI infusion thereafter. After surgery, SC insulin therapy should be restarted when the patient has recommenced their normal diet; the GKI infusion should continue for at least until an hour after the first SC insulin dose is administered.

3. Diabetic children, who are scheduled to undergo minor elective surgery on an afternoon operating list, should be allowed to have a normal breakfast and their morning insulin dose

(i.e. two-thirds of the short-acting component should be given as Actrapid®). Upon arrival in the morning, their capillary blood glucose levels should be checked, and they should be encouraged to maintain a 'clear fluid' oral intake to avoid dehydration until two hours prior to surgery, after which, they are completely starved. It is only at this time that hourly blood glucose monitoring will be required to ensure normoglycaemia until surgery is commenced.

15. Answers: 1-D; 2-F; 3-C

The TNM Classification of Malignant Tumours (TNM) is a staging system for solid tumours that was devised by Pierre Denoix between 1943 and 1952. It uses the size and extension of the primary tumour, its lymphatic involvement, and the presence of metastasis to classify the progression of cancer:

- T describes the tumour size and adjacent tissue invasion
- N describes the involvement of locoregional lymph nodes
- M describes the presence of distant metastasis

1. The TNM classification system for renal cancer is as follows:

Primary tumour:

T1: ≤7 cm in diameter; confined to kidney

T2: >7 cm in diameter; confined to kidney

T3: involvement of perinephric fat, renal vein, or the inferior vena cava

T4: tumour extending outside pararenal fascia

Regional lymph nodes:

N0: no locoregional lymph node involvement

N1: involvement of single lymph node

N2: involvement of two or more lymph nodes

Distant metastasis:

M0: no evidence of distant metastasis

M1: distant metastasis present (e.g. to lungs, bone, brain)

The patient in this scenario has a 9 cm diameter (T2) renal tumour with two positive nodes (N2) and no evidence of distant metastasis (M0), resulting in a tumour stage of T2N2M0.

2. The TNM classification system for malignant melanoma is as follows:

Primary tumour:

Tis: melanoma in situ

T1: ≤1.0 mm in diameter

T2: 1.01–2.0 mm in diameter

T3: 2.01–4.0 mm in diameter

T4: >4.0 mm in diameter

Regional lymph nodes:

N0: no locoregional lymph node involvement

N1: involvement of single lymph node

N2: involvement of 2–3 lymph nodes

N3: involvement of ≥ 4 lymph nodes

Distant metastasis:

M0: no evidence of distant metastasis

M1a: metastasis to skin, subcutaneous or distant lymph nodes; normal serum LDH

M1b: lung metastases present; normal serum LDH

M1c: distant metastasis present; elevated serum LDH

The patient in this scenario has a 3 mm diameter (T3) malignant melanoma with two positive nodes (N2) and no evidence of distant metastasis (M0), resulting in a tumour stage of T3N2M0.

3. The TNM classification system for breast cancer is as follows:

Primary tumour:

Tis: carcinoma in situ

T1: ≤2 cm in diameter

T2: >2 cm but ≤ 5 cm in diameter

T3: > 5 cm in diameter

T4: any size with direct extension to the chest wall and/or the skin (ulceration, peau d'orange)

Regional lymph nodes:

N0: no locoregional lymph node involvement

N1: involvement of mobile, ipsilateral axillary nodes

N2: involvement of ipsilateral axillary nodes that are fixed to one another, or to other structures

N3: involvement of ipsilateral internal mammary nodes

Distant metastasis:

M0: no evidence of distant metastasis

M1: distant metastasis present (e.g. to ipsilateral supraclavicular nodes)

The patient in this scenario has a 3 cm diameter (T2) breast tumour with the involvement of mobile, ipsilateral axillary nodes (N1)s, and no evidence of distant metastasis (M0), resulting in a tumour stage of T2N1M0.

16. Answers: 1-B; 2-H; 3-I

1. In this scenario, the patient demonstrates signs of benign prostatic hyperplasia, which has resulted in bladder outflow obstruction and chronic urinary retention, with evidence of renal impairment. In cases of progressive prostate enlargement, the resultant bladder outflow obstruction and rise in bladder volume results in an increase in intravesical pressure. This pressure is transmitted backwards via the ureters, causing hydronephrosis and progressive renal parenchymal damage. Although prompt catheterization is indicated in these patients, often producing significant symptomatic relief, doing so often produces a massive diuresis. It is therefore vital to monitor these patients' fluid and electrolyte balance closely to ensure haemodynamic stability, as well as any improvements in renal function.

2. An intra-abdominal pressure of over 10–12 mmHg (i.e. intra-abdominal hypertension) is associated with reduced perfusion to the abdominal organs. Abdominal compartment syndrome

is said to occur when intra-abdominal pressures exceed 20 mmHg, leading to impairing pulmonary, cardiovascular, renal, and gastrointestinal dysfunction, and potentially progressing to multiple organ dysfunction syndrome, and death. Such patients often present with a fall in urine output and increased ventilator requirements. Approximately 30% of all surgical patients on the Intensive Care Unit develop intra-abdominal hypertension, which in itself, is an independent risk factor for mortality. In patients who are suspected to have intra-abdominal hypertension, the intra-abdominal pressure may be measured by connecting a pressure transducer to a urinary catheter. A timely decompression with re-laparotomy may be vital in restoring organ function to these patients.

3. It is important to remember that pyelonephritis in the presence of an obstructed urinary tract is an urological emergency, due to the tendency of such patients to develop systemic sepsis and deteriorate rapidly. Early renal ultrasonography is therefore vital in patients with suspected pyelonephritis, to exclude the presence of concurrent hydronephrosis. In the event of an infected, obstructed kidney resulting in acute renal failure, an emergency percutaneous nephrostomy is the treatment of choice. These patients should also receive intravenous antibiotic therapy and fluid resuscitation. If further imaging suggests the obstruction to be secondary to advanced pelvic malignancy, double J-stents ureteric may be palliatively inserted, and nephrostomies avoided (i.e. due to the long-term risks of infection and general discomfort associated with nephrostomies.)

17. Answers: 1-F; 2-H; 3-C

1. This patient's history and examination findings are consistent with intermittent claudication. He is most likely to benefit from a left-to-right femoro-femoral bypass graft. An alternative to this would be an ilio-femoral bypass from the external iliac artery, which may provide better flow dynamics and avoid a femoral incision (i.e. which would confer a higher risk of wound infection than an abdominal wound would do). Although angioplasty (and stenting) is usually the first step in the invasive management of such disease, the long occlusion in this case would preclude this management option. An aorto-bifemoral bypass would involve major vascular reconstruction and, as such, is unnecessary in this case as the aorta and left iliac systems are not significantly diseased.

2. This arteriopathic gentleman has occluded both of his bypass grafts, with no option for salvage remaining. It must be emphasized to the patient that he is at serious risk of losing both of his legs, and that immediate smoking cessation is essential. He may benefit from a lumbar sympathectomy, which involves the excision of the 2nd and 3rd lumbar ganglia, and may be performed laparoscopically. The indications for lumbar sympathectomy include critical limb ischaemia (characterized by pain at rest), digital ischaemia and ischaemic ulceration. Unfortunately, lumbar sympathectomy often does not produce significant symptomatic improvement, and any benefit derived from it may only be temporary.

3. This patient's claudication symptoms are clearly related to her aorto-iliac occlusive disease. In this case, an 'extra-anatomic' bypass is indicated to restore perfusion to both femoral arteries. Although aorto-bifemoral bypass grafts may offer better long-term patency, this patient's severely impaired cardiovascular status places her at high risk of mortality and morbidity following such major surgery. Regardless of the utility of each procedure, it is important to consider the overall benefit (versus risk) that this patient is likely to obtain from surgery, as her exercise tolerance may not actually improve after the operation (e.g. due to her breathlessness). Furthermore, claudication is not a life- or limb-threatening condition and so the best initial management would comprise best medical care alone.

18. Answers: 1-G; 2-C; 3-B

1. This patient has sustained bilateral mandibular fractures, which typically occur as the result of a direct blow to the jaw during a fall, assault or sports injury. Unilateral trauma often produces an ipsilateral mandibular body fracture and a contralateral subcondylar fracture, while a high impact to the symphysis produces a symphyseal fracture and bilateral subcondylar fractures. It is vital to exclude damage to the cervical spine in such patients. Examination should account for abnormalities in facial contour, as well as the shape, tenderness, swelling, and presence of lacerations or haematomas of the mandibular region. Mandibular movements and malocclusion should be assessed, and loose or missing teeth should be accounted for. Paraesthesia (or anaesthesia) of the chin may indicate mandibular nerve damage (i.e. at the inferior alveolar nerve or mental nerve) – this should be documented together with any damage to the marginal mandibular nerve branch of the facial nerve. Importantly, spasm of the masticatory muscles may produce trismus, impairing examination and distracting any fractures. In this patient, posterior displacement of the tongue, potentially leading to obstruction of the oropharynx and airway compromise, requires that the airway be secured urgently (i.e. with intubation and ventilation), after which, CT imaging should be performed to delineate the extent of the maxillofacial injury.

2. This patient has sustained an extradural haemorrhage, which commonly results from trauma to the temporoparietal region—especially at the thin pterion—causing a rupture of one of the meningeal arteries between the dura and the skull (i.e. most commonly, the middle meningeal artery). The patient is often a young adult (since the dura becomes increasingly adherent to the skull with age), sustaining a concussion that may be followed by transient recovery of consciousness for minutes or hours before the onset of drowsiness and subsequent coma (i.e. the 'lucid interval'). Clinical features of raised intracranial pressure in these patients include an ipsilateral, dilated pupil on the side of the expanding lesion; a bilateral III nerve palsy (as tentorial herniation occurs); progressive contralateral hemiplegia, nausea, vomiting, etc. A CT scan of the head is mandatory in such presentations, and often demonstrates a peripheral, biconvex (due the dura being pushed inwards), high-attenuation lesion (indicating fresh haemorrhage due to the early nature of such presentations). After identifying the site of haemorrhage on CT imaging, the management of extradural haemorrhage involves complete evacuation through a 'horse shoe' craniotomy flap. In cases of rapid clinical deterioration, temporary relief may be attained by means of a burr hole and craniectomy, positioned centrally over the haematoma. The overall prognosis depends on the patient's GCS prior to surgery, with mortality rates as high as 20% in comatose patients.

3. This patient has sustained a subdural haematoma, which typically occurs in elderly patients following minor head trauma, resulting in rupture of the cortical bridging veins. These veins serve to connect the cerebral venous system to the intradural venous sinuses, and lie relatively exposed within the subdural space. Predisposing factors include cerebral atrophy (e.g. in the elderly) and low cerebrospinal fluid pressure after shunting (e.g. for longstanding hydrocephalus), both of which tend to stretch the bridging veins; alcoholism; and impaired clotting function. Clinical features tend to develop more gradually than those from extradural haemorrhage, as the bleeding is of low-pressure venous origin. They include fluctuating conscious levels (i.e. with gradual-onset headache, memory loss, personality changes, confusion and drowsiness) and focal neurological signs (e.g. ipsilateral hemiparesis, a false localizing sign; and aphasia, in left-sided lesions). A CT scan of the head is mandatory in such presentations, and often demonstrates a peripheral, crescentic (due to containment of the haematoma within the non-stretchable dura), low-attenuation lesion (indicating clotted blood, due to the subacute or delayed nature of such presentations). In adults with depressed conscious levels, the haematoma may be evacuated via 2–3 burr holes, followed by saline irrigation of the cavity, and nursing in the head-down position

to prevent re-accumulation. Adults with normal conscious levels may be managed conservatively (e.g. with steroids over several weeks). In infants, subdural haematomas may be evacuated via the anterior fontanelle by repeated needle aspiration; while persistent collections may be amenable to subdural peritoneal shunting.

19. Answers: 1-G; 2-F; 3-D; 4-I

1. Complex internal trauma can often be concealed in young and fit individuals, who are able to physiologically compensate for systemic insults to a greater degree than older patients. In trauma care, the standard primary and secondary surveys need to be performed, together with immediate resuscitation of the patient. In this case, blood at the external urethral meatus is highly suggestive of urethral injury. A retrograde urethrogram should therefore be performed prior to attempting urethral catheterization. If this confirms urethral injury, a suprapubic catheter should be inserted to drain the bladder before further evaluation of the injury, to determine if urethral reconstruction is indicated.

2. This patient has developed acute renal failure secondary to urinary tract obstruction from his advanced prostate malignancy. The fact that the patient remains oliguric following urethral catheterization suggests either an intrinsic renal injury (i.e. from longstanding urinary retention secondary to bladder outflow obstruction), or more likely, occlusion of the ureteric orifices by the locally advanced prostate tumour. This is a urological emergency and the immediate priority would be to relieve the urinary tract obstruction, to minimize ongoing renal damage. This should be achieved via bilateral percutaneous nephrostomies, after confirmation of bilateral hydronephrosis and hydroureter on ultrasound imaging. If urethral catheterization is initially impossible (e.g. due to a stenosed prostatic urethra), suprapubic catheterization may be attempted before an intravenous pyelogram (or CT urogram) is performed.

3. As with the patient in Scenario 2, the immediate priority in this situation would be to relieve the urinary tract obstruction, in order to minimize any ongoing renal injury. It is vital to consider this patient's past urological history, as his obstructed single kidney should not undergo percutaneous nephrostomy tube placement in the first instance, due to the risk of renal damage associated with this procedure. A retrograde ureteric stent insertion should first be attempted instead, as this will not only relieve the obstruction but also ensure a degree of ureteric patency in the near future. This patient may concurrently require analgesia and selective alpha-blockers (e.g. Tamsulosin) to ameliorate his ureteric stone disease, and further definitive imaging to assist its management.

4. This patient's history and examination findings are consistent with acute urinary tract obstruction secondary to clot retention. Although establishing the cause of the patient's haematuria is essential, the immediate priority would be to relieve the urinary tract obstruction. This should be attempted with a three-way catheter to drain the bladder, and for subsequent bladder irrigation. It is important to carefully monitor the patient's urine output and remember that absolute anuria in a catheterized patient is almost always due to catheter obstruction rather than an intrinsic renal problem. This should prompt flushing of the catheter before any further investigations are undertaken.

20. Answers: 1-C; 2-F; 3-H

1. Infantile pyloric stenosis affects 1 in 400 neonates, demonstrating both a male preponderance (M:F = 4:1) and a familial component, and typically affecting the first-born child. Although previously believed to be congenital, the condition is now considered to be acquired at an early stage, manifesting in the first 3–6 weeks of life. It has been associated with Turner's

syndrome, oesophageal atresia and phenylketonuria. The pathology stems from a failure of relaxation of the pyloric sphincter (i.e. possibly from a deficiency in nitric oxide synthase in the myenteric plexus), resulting in intense hypertrophy of the adjacent pyloric muscle. The classic symptom is projectile, non-bilious vomiting (i.e. as the obstruction is proximal to the sphincter of Oddi) in a child who remains hungry and eats immediately after vomiting. Examination often reveals a dehydrated, emaciated child, with visible peristalsis of the dilated stomach in the epigastric region. The majority of affected infants will demonstrate a palpable olive-shaped pyloric mass in the right hypochondrium, especially after the child is giving a drink, or 'test feed'. A barium meal may reveal delayed gastric emptying; a dilated stomach and a narrowed, attenuated pyloric canal (i.e. the 'string sign'). Initial blood tests may reveal a hypokalaemic, hypochloraemic metabolic alkalosis, which should be addressed (together with the dehydration) by careful fluid resuscitation. Following this, the surgical treatment of choice is Ramstedt's pyloromyotomy.

2. Congenital duodenal atresia, which involves the absence or obstruction of a functional duodenum, may be secondary to a complete absence of the duodenum, a fibrous band, a diaphragm, or a partial diaphragm. The anomaly most commonly occurs at the junction between the foregut and midgut. The common bile duct usually enters the duodenum proximal to the obstruction, leading to bilious vomiting (i.e. in contrast to the non-bilious vomiting in hypertrophic pyloric stenosis, when the obstruction is proximal to the sphincter of Oddi). The pathology usually results from the failure of the duodenum to epithelialize at five weeks of gestation, followed by vacuolization and recanalization by week eight. At birth, profuse vomiting may be noted with visible abdominal distension. Similar symptoms may manifest with oesophageal atresia (although this results in choking, rather than vomiting); pyloric stenosis (although this typically involves non-bilious vomitus, a palpable abdominal mass on test feed, and a later presentation at 3–6 weeks from birth); and congenital intestinal obstruction (although abdominal radiography will demonstrate air throughout the obstructed bowel, in contrast with duodenal atresia, which will feature only gastric and proximal duodenal dilatation). Investigations must include measurements of electrolytes and acid-base balance, plain abdominal radiography (potentially revealing the 'double bubble' sign of duodenal obstruction), and a barium meal. After ensuring that all metabolic parameters are stable, the surgical management involves forming a duodenojejunostomy and resection of the atresic bowel. A recognised association exists between congenial duodenal atresia and Down's syndrome.

3. A tracheoesophageal fistula (TOF) refers to an abnormal connection between the trachea and oesophagus, typically resulting from a failure of normal development. The majority of TOF variants involve a blind-ending oesophagus, with fistulation between the distal oesophagus and trachea. TOF may rarely involve a communication between an intact oesophagus and the trachea (i.e. H-type TOF). Infants with TOF are usually symptomatic from birth, presenting with postprandial choking and cyanosis, recurrent aspiration pneumonia (i.e. due to milk and other feeds passing from the oesophagus into the airways), and abdominal distension (i.e. if a connection exists between the oesophagus, trachea and stomach). After radiographic or endoscopic confirmation of TOF, the initial management involves rehydration and correction of any electrolyte or glycaemic imbalances, together with the treatment of aspiration pneumonia, and nursing with a tube to provide continual suction drainage of the oesophageal pouch. The definitive surgical correction of TOF involves an end-to-end anastomosis through a right thoracotomy (in the bed of the fifth rib). The azygos vein is then doubly ligated and divided, and the mediastinal pleura incised. Any fistulae encountered are divided at their entrance into the trachea and sewn shut, followed by mobilization of the proximal pouch and establishing the end-to-end anastomosis.

21. Answers: 1-I; 2-C; 3-H

1. Testicular teratomas are derived from multi-potent cells that contain tissue from all three testicular germ layers, exhibiting a wide range of differentiation. They commonly secrete human chorionic gonadotropin and/or alpha-feto protein, which can be measured in the serum and used as tumour markers. Chemotherapy with platinum-based combinations forms the mainstay of treatment for testicular teratoma, offering an overall 5-year survival of up to 95%. Examples of such platinum-containing agents include cisplatin and carboplatin, which both offer better side-effect profiles and recurrence rates than radiotherapy does (note that teratomas are less radiosensitive than seminomas). In contrast, seminomas are testicular tumours that are derived from seminiferous tubular cells and secrete human chorionic gonadotropin (but not typically alpha-feto protein). They are solid, slow-growing tumours that are exquisitely radiosensitive, unlike teratomas. While teratomas occur most commonly between the ages of 20–30 years, seminomas usually occur in the 30–40 year age group.

2. The management of colonic carcinoma includes surgical resection (e.g. colectomy with en bloc clearance of regional lymph nodes for non-metastatic colonic tumours; or resection of metastatic disease and colectomy in metastatic tumours that are deemed to be resectable). Chemotherapy (e.g. with 5-fluorouracil or 5-FU) may be used after surgery for high-risk stage II and stage III colonic tumours, and before surgery for resectable metastatic disease. Current evidence supports the use of adjuvant chemotherapy in metastatic disease, as it increases the 3-year disease-free survival rate to 10–12% in patients with stage III colorectal cancer. It is important to remember that for colonic cancer, the response to radiotherapy is limited by the challenge of directing the therapeutic radiation at the tumour without damaging surrounding structures (e.g. the bladder). In comparison, patients with inoperable rectal cancer may be managed palliatively with both radiotherapy and cytotoxic chemotherapy. Further treatment with adjuvant chemotherapy should be considered after surgery for high-risk stage II and stage III (Dukes C) rectal cancer.

3. Although up to 70% of patients with small cell lung cancer (SCLC) have extensive disease at the time of diagnosis, approximately 80% of patients respond to combination chemotherapy due to the high chemosensitivity of SCLC. Platinum-based combination chemotherapy may induce temporary remission and increase life expectancy in these patients. In conjunction with chemotherapy, NICE recommends that thoracic irradiation should be used to improve survival in patients with limited disease; and after chemotherapy in extensive disease, if a good response from chemotherapy is observed. In order to reduce the risk of brain metastases, prophylactic radiotherapy may also be used in patients who respond to chemotherapy. It must be remembered that in most cases of SCLC, treatment is palliative (i.e. palliative chemotherapy for tumour debulking and extending survival; palliative radiotherapy to ease pain or bronchial obstruction; pleurodesis for recurrent pleural effusions; and palliative endoscopic laser therapy for obstructive lesions of the large airways).

22. Answers: 1-F; 2-A; 3-D

Thoracotomy is a major surgical procedure involving an incision into the thoracic pleural space to access certain intrathoracic structures. The choice of incision depends on the underlying pathology, the site (e.g. lung, chest wall, oesophagus), and the experience of the surgeon. Thoracoscopic (e.g. video-assisted thoracic surgery or VATS) approaches are now used widely for pneumothorax and pleural effusion surgery.

After thoracotomy, the importance of adequate postoperative analgesia is emphasized by the high probability of inadequate ventilation (i.e. secondary to pain), which may lead to atelectasis or pneumonia. Many surgical units use epidural analgesia for all thoracotomies; an alternative is a paravertebral catheter placed behind the pleura at the end of surgery.

In addition to postoperative respiratory failure and infection, thoracotomy may be complicated by pneumothorax, haemothorax, pleural effusion, and surgical emphysema. In an attempt to avoid such complications, chest drains are placed in nearly all thoracotomy operations. It is important for clinicians to ensure that these tubes remain unoccluded by fibrinous material or clot in the postoperative period.

1. The posterolateral thoracotomy involves an incision through an intercostal space on the back, and is one of the most common approaches to the thoracic cavity. It is the approach of choice for pulmonary resection (e.g. pneumonectomy and lobectomy) and is also used for oesophageal resection, and, occasionally, cardiac surgery. On the left side, it provides good exposure of the aortic arch and descending aorta, and on the right side, the distal trachea and superior vena cava. It also allows optimal exposure of mediastinal and hilar structures (e.g. major pulmonary vessels) and the hemidiaphragm on each side. It must be noted that although this incision heals well, it takes considerable time to open and close the thorax with this approach, largely due to the meticulous dissection required.

2. A bilateral anterolateral thoractomy combined with transverse sternotomy results in the 'clamshell' incision—the largest incision commonly employed in thoracic surgery. It is used to gain quick access to the superior mediastinum, and provides excellent exposure of both pleural spaces, which is beneficial in emergent scenarios such as this. Its main indication in elective surgery is for bilateral lung transplantation but it can also be used for bilateral pulmonary metastasectomy. The considerable postoperative pain that results from the procedure necessitates epidural analgesia, when circumstances permit. The procedure involves using bone cutters to divide the manubrium to the level of the manubriosternal joint. The intercostal muscles within the second intercostal space are divided to the mid-axillary line, where the rib is divided on each side, thus forming the so-called 'clamshell' opening.

3. The median sternotomy is the most common incision utilized by cardiothoracic surgeons in the UK, and gives excellent exposure to the heart, great vessels, and both hemidiaphragms. It also allows for excellent exposure for thymoma surgery, and is occasionally used for bilateral lung procedures (e.g. lung volume reduction surgery). However, the median sternotomy affords limited exposure of the pleural space and the anterior hilar structures. Its advantages include less compromise of pulmonary function, and less postoperative pain, compared to any standard thoracotomy. During such access, a single-lumen endotracheal tube is utilized in all situations except when lung surgery is involved (i.e. when single-lung ventilation anaesthesia with a double-lumen endobronchial tube may be used.)

23. Answers: 1-A; 2-D; 3-J

1. Kaplan–Meier survival curves (i.e. 'life curves') are used to represent outcomes that are timed to an event. They are widely used in survival analysis, and they represent the proportion of the study population that remains surviving at successive times. The curve begins at 1 (or 100%) at time 0 (i.e. when all patients are presumed to be alive) and tails down in a stepwise fashion whenever an event occurs, until 0, when all patients are dead. As the number of subjects in each intervention group decreases over time, the curves are considered to be more precise on the left (i.e. earlier periods) rather than the right (i.e. later periods). To account for this, the relative risk of the event of interest over the entire study period should be weighted for the number of subjects available over time; this weighted relative risk is known as the hazard ratio.

2. The negative predictive value (NPV) refers to the post-test probability of a negative test result eventually leading to a negative diagnosis. It answers the question, 'If a patient has a negative test result, what is the probability that he/she does not actually have the disease?' The NPV is calculated as: [true negatives / (false negatives + true negatives) x 100%] In contrast, the positive predictive value (PPV) refers to the post-test probability of a positive test result eventually leading to a positive diagnosis. It should also be noted that the 'sensitivity' of a test refers to the test's ability to identify positive results (i.e. the rate of true positives); while 'specificity' refers to the ability of a test to identify negative results (i.e. the rate of true negatives).

3. The null hypothesis is a formal statement that no difference exists between sample groups (e.g. a placebo group versus a treatment group), or that there is no association between the risk indicator and the outcomes variables. If the null hypothesis is found to be true, it may be concluded that any result is due to chance or random factors. If the null hypothesis is rejected, there may be evidence of a difference between treatment groups, or an association between risk indicator and outcome variables. A type 1 error (alpha), as in this scenario, results from incorrectly rejecting a true null hypothesis (i.e. producing a false positive result). In contrast, a type 2 error (beta) results from incorrectly accepting a false null hypothesis (i.e. producing a false negative result). If a type 2 error is known, the power of a study may be calculated from: (1 − probability of type 2 error).

24. Answers: 1-G; 2-D; 3-B; 4-C

It is vital for surgeons to have a sound understanding of the principles and practice of diathermy, and how to avoid its potential complications. The principles of surgical diathermy dictate that when an electrical current passes through a conductor, some of its energy is dissipated as heat. The amount of this heating effect depends on the intensity and waveform of the current, the electrical properties of the tissues through which the current passes, and the relative size of the two electrodes. Although mains electricity is of 50 Hz frequency and is capable of producing intense muscle and nerve activation, diathermy electrical frequency ranges from 300 kHz to 3 MHz, and therefore does not activate these tissues. Monopolar diathermy involves the use of an electrical plate stuck onto the patient (i.e. the indifferent electrode)—current flows between this and the active diathermy electrode. A localized heating effect is produced at the tip of the active electrode, which has a surface area of an order of magnitude less than that of the indifferent electrode, allowing minimal heating effect to be induced at the latter. In contrast, bipolar diathermy combines two active electrodes within the instrument (e.g. diathermy forceps)— current therefore flows between the tips of these electrodes (and any tissue between them), and not through the rest of the patient. The main effects of diathermy on tissues include coagulation (i.e. cell death by dehydration and protein denaturation, to seal off blood vessels), fulguration (i.e. a higher-voltage destructive coagulation of tissues with carbonization and charring), and cutting (i.e. when sufficient heat is applied to tissues to cause water to explode into steam, to separate effectively divide tissues). Some of the major complications of diathermy are described as follows:

1. Sparks from the active diathermy electrode may ignite any volatile or inflammable gas within the operation theatre. Alcohol-based skin preparations may ignite if they are allowed to pool on/ around the patient. In addition, diathermy should be avoided in the presence of potentially explosive gases, including those which may occur naturally in the colon (e.g. methane and hydrogen), especially after certain forms of bowel preparation (e.g. mannitol). Caution must especially be exercised in endoscopic diathermy of the large bowel (e.g. when diathermy is used to coagulate and seal the base of snared polyps), during which an explosion may cause colonic rupture.

2. Although most modern cardiac pacemakers are designed to be inhibited by high-frequency interference (i.e. so that the patient receives no pacing stimulation when diathermy is active), diathermy currents may still affect pacemaker function by conduction (e.g. when diathermy is used in the thorax or upper abdomen). Certain demand pacemakers may revert to the fixed pacing rate, making it important for the anaesthetist to have an appropriate magnet available to reset the pacemaker, if necessary. In most patients with pacemakers, it is therefore advisable to use bipolar diathermy whenever possible. If monopolar diathermy must be used, the electrical plate should be sited as far away from the pacemaker site as possible to avoid inadvertent conductance of current to the heart or the pacemaker site.

3. Capacitance coupling is the phenomenon by which a capacitor is created by having an insulator sandwiched between two conducting electrodes. If a metal laparoscopic port has a diathermy hook passed through it, the insulation of the diathermy hook acts as the sandwiched insulator, and by means of electromagnetic induction, the diathermy current within the hook may induce a current within the metal port, which may potentially damage intraperitoneal structures and other structures that it passes through. Although current is usually dissipated from the metal port through the abdominal wall, this dissipation cannot occur if a plastic cuff is used, significantly increasing the risk of capacitance coupling. Metal ports should therefore never be used with plastic cuffs; nonetheless, injuries due to capacitance coupling are becoming rarer due to the increasing use of fully-plastic ports.

4. The heat produced from diathermy is maximal at the point of greatest current density. Although this would normally be at the tip of the active electrode, if current is channelled up a narrow path or pedicle, enough heat may be generated within this space to coagulate the adjacent tissues. This may prove highly injurious in certain situations (e.g. coagulation of narrow appendages, such as the penis in a child undergoing circumcision; or coagulation of the spermatic cord, when the active electrode is applied to the testis). In such situations, the surgeon must avoid the use of diathermy if possible, or use only bipolar diathermy (i.e. to restrict the path of the current), if required.

INDEX

Key: ■ denotes question, ■ denotes answer

abdominal aortic aneurysm (AAA) 137
abdominal compartment syndrome 142–3
abdominal haemorrhage 95
abdominal migraine 66
abdominal pain 49
abdominoperineal resection 60, 98
ABL (Abelson murine leukaemia) viral oncogene 96
achalasia cardia 93
Acinetobacter baumannii 132
acute haemolytic transfusion reactions 60
acute respiratory distress syndrome (ARDS) 31
adrenal tumours 67
adrenalectomy 51
adrenaline (intramuscular) 98
alkylating agents, DNA damage 59
alpha-blockade, phenoxybenzamine 67
Alvarado score 65
aminoglycoside antibiotics 29
anaemia
    classification 64
    iron deficiency 63
    secondary to menorrhagia 42
anaphylaxis
    drug-induced 97
    transfusion reactions 60
anastrozole 105
androgen receptor antagonist
        (cyproterone acetate) 105
ankylosing spondylitis 20
anti-diabetics, oral 140
antibiotics 96
    aminoglycosides 29
    anti-tumour antibiotics 60
    broad-spectrum 32
    cephalosporins 29
    fluoroquinolones 29
    prophylaxis 140
anticoagulation, contraindications for 30
antimetabolites, classification 59
aortic dissection, traumatic 59
aorto-bifemoral bypass 143
appendicitis
    acute 94
    Alvarado score 65

aromatase inhibitors 32
    anastrozole 105
arterial blood gases 100
arthritis
    rheumatoid arthritis 30, 63
    sexually-acquired reactive 21
assessment, see trauma assessment and triage
atelectasis 24, 95
atrial fibrillation 43
    new-onset 31
audit cycle 139
Auerbach's plexus 105
Austin Moore prosthesis 28
autoclave 34
avascular necrosis of femoral head 28

'bamboo spine' 20
Barrett's oesophagus 101
Battle's sign 134
beta-2 microglobin 101
bile duct injury 137
Billroth I/II procedures 69
bisphosphonates 69
blood products 42
Bolam test 28
bone pain, metastatic 69
bowel cancer 42, 43
bowel obstruction 58
bowel surgery, anastomotic leakage 58, 63
breast abscess 133
    Staphylococcus aureus infection 133, 135
breast cancer 105
    adjuvant hormone therapy 32
    TNM classification 142
Breslow thickness 21
bronchopleural fistula 94
Burkitt's lymphoma 96
burns 24
    skin loss 5
bursitis 57
bypass
    aorto-bifemoral bypass 143
    femoro-femoral bypass graft 143
    femoropopliteal bypass 51

C-myc gene 96
calcitonin 101
capacitance coupling 150
cardiac failure 95
cardiac tamponade 95
cardiogenic shock 97
carotid endarterectomy 44
case reports, case series 63
case work-up 122
catecholamines 67
cauda equina syndrome 20
cellulitis 95, 135
cephalosporin 132
cervical cancer, radioactive sources 33
cervical lymphadenopathy 94
chemoradiation therapy 60
    preoperative 60
chemotherapy
    adjuvant 32
    palliative 26
cholecystectomy 46
chromogranin A 101
Clark's index 21
clinical audit 139
clinical decision-making 6, 11, 17, 18, 41, 45, 75, 78, 81,
    87, 124, 128
clinical governance 120, 139
clinical reasoning 43
clinical trials
    clinical outcome 26
    evidence and guidelines 44
    strength of evidence 62
Clostridium difficile, pseudomembranous colitis 32
Clostridium perfringens 25
closures (sutures) 18, 33
coagulation 13
    anticoagulation 30
cohort studies 63
colitis 45, 135
    Clostridium difficile 135
    fulminating 56, 68
    inflammatory/infectious 56
    ischaemic 56
    pseudomembranous 32, 132, 134
    ulcerative colitis 28, 56, 63, 68
colonic carcinoma 61, 147
    metastatic bone pain 69
colorectal cancer 29, 147
    Dukes' staging 25
colovesical fistula 63
common peroneal nerve injuries 57
competence 28
    Gillick 97, 99
    incompetence 28
compression bandaging 96
consent issues 10, 28, 77, 80, 97–8
    child 97, 99

decision against medical advice 99
    senior attending clinician 99
continuing professional development 139
continuous hyper-fractionated accelerated radiotherapy
    (CHART) 18, 33
continuous positive airway pressure (CPAP) ventilation 138
correlation coefficient 26
critical care 48, 76, 82, 112, 116, 119, 123
Crohn's disease 46, 68, 132
crutches 23
cyclical vomiting syndrome 66
cytochrome P450 29

Dance's sign 94
deep vein thrombosis (DVT) 13, 24, 30, 97
dermatofibroma 131
diabetes mellitus 27, 37
    perioperative care 121
diagnostic laparoscopy 103
diaphragmatic splinting 24
diarrhoea, enterotoxin-related 32
diathermy 130
    explosion 149
    heat channelling 150
differential diagnosis 8, 15, 17, 47, 49, 53, 73, 85
diverticular abscess 63
diverticular disease 49, 61, 68
DNA damage, alkylating agents 59
dobutamine 98
Down's syndrome 146
drains 107–8
    use of 91
drug-induced anaphylaxis 97
duodenal atresia, congenital 146
duodenal ulcers 69
dysphagia 92, 98

elderly patients, aromatase inhibitors 32
electrolytes 65
    child 65
embolism 13
emergency laparotomy 45
endometrial cancer 105
endoscopic retrograde cholangiopancreatography
    (ERCP) 137
endovascular aneurysm repair (EVAR) 137
enteral nutrition 26, 98
erysipelas 135
    Streptococcus pyogenes 135
ESBL-related urosepsis 140
ethylene oxide 33
evidence
    and guidelines 44
    strength of 62
extended right hemicolectomy 98
extended-spectrum beta-lactamase (ESBL)-producing
    organisms 140

extracorporeal membrane oxygenation (ECMO) 138–9
extradural haematoma 134
extradural haemorrhage 144

factor V Leiden mutation 30
faecal contamination 29, 32, 136
fat embolism syndrome (FES) 31
feeding
  enteral 26, 98
  parenteral 101–2
  PEG 26, 97
feeding jejunostomy 102
femoral neck fractures 28
femoro-femoral bypass graft 143
femoropopliteal bypass 51
femur, avascular necrosis 28
fetus, consent issues 28
fibrous histiocytoma 131
fistulas, causes 58
fluid requirements
  hypovolaemia 65
  paediatrics 65
  Parkland formula 25
  therapy 48
focused assessment with sonography for trauma (FAST)
    scan 103
foot drop 57, 58
fractures
  classification 106
  femoral neck 28
  Gustilo classification 106, 107
  mandibular 143
  reduction 107
  skull 134
  tibial 107
Froment's sign 23, 136

Garden classification, femoral neck fractures 28
gastrectomy 26
gastric cancer 67–8
  adenocarcinoma 52
gastric ulcers 69
gastro-oesophageal reflux disease (GORD) 93, 103
gastrointestinal bleeding
  lower 41, 42
  upper 30
gastrointestinal disease 71–91, 110, 118
  diagnosis 35
gastrointestinal perforations 69
gastrojejunostomy 69
general anaesthesia 44
gentamicin 29
Gillick competence 97, 99
glaucoma, acute closed-angle 30
glutaraldehyde, sterilization of equipment 33
goserelin 105
Gram-positive cocci 31, 32

Gurd and Wilson criteria, fat embolism syndrome 31
gut ischaemia 31

haemochromatosis 61
Haemophilus influenzae 67
haemorrhage
  abdominal 95
  extradural 144
  haemothorax 39
  retroperitoneal 103
haemostasis 42
haemothorax, massive 39
Hartmann's procedure 91
  sigmoid tumour 29, 63
head and neck surgery 2, 109
Helicobacter pylori 67–8
hemicolectomy, right 98
heparin 97
hereditary spherocytosis 63
hernias
  direct inguinal 99, 103
  femoral 99, 102
  incisional 91
  indirect inguinal 102
  repair with mesh fixation 46, 100
  Richter's 102
  truss support 100
hip replacement 37, 42
  Austin Moore prosthesis 28
  hemiarthroplasty 28
Hirschsprung's disease 105
history, examination and assessment 115, 127
hormone therapy, adjuvant 32
Hutchinson's melanotic freckle 22
hydronephrosis 27
hypercoagulable states 30
hypertension, intra-abdominal 142–3
hypovolaemic shock 42
hypoxia 136

ileal pouch-anal anastomosis 63
incisions 54, 68–9, 129
  clamshell 148
  median sternotomy 148
infantile pyloric stenosis 106, 145–6
inferior vena cava filters 30
inflammatory bowel disease 35, 131
insulin therapy 140
intermittent claudication 143
intermittent positive pressure ventilation (IPPV) 138
interstitial oedema, Kerley B lines 95
intestinal obstruction 58
intra-abdominal hypertension 142–3
intraocular pressure reduction 30
intraoperative care 12
intraperitoneal abscess 31
intussusception 94

inverse ratio ventilation (IRV) 133
investigations 43, 62, 126
    planning 83, 118
iron deficiency anaemia 63
iron overload 61
ischiorectal abscess 92
Ivor Lewis procedure 99, 104

jaundice 137–8
jejunostomy feeding 99

Kaplan–Meier survival curves 26, 148
Karydakis technique 106
keratoacanthoma 23
keratoderma blenorrhagica 21
Kerley B lines 95
Kessler technique, modified 106
Kruskal–Wallis test 26

lactic acidosis, metformin-associated 140
Lanz incision 69
laparotomy
    emergency 45
    faecal contamination 29, 136
large bowel obstruction 29, 45
lentigo maligna melanoma 22
Lewis–Tanner procedure 26, 99, 104
limb ischaemia 143
Li–Fraumeni syndrome 95
loop colostomy 63
lower back pain 52
lumbar disc herniation (prolapse) 20
lumbar puncture 134
lumbar spondylolisthesis 20
lumbar sympathectomy 143
Lund and Browder chart 24
lung cancer, treatment with CHART 33
lupus vulgaris 131

McBurney's incision 69
magnetic resonance cholangiopancreatography
    (MRCP) 137
malignant melanoma 21
mandibular fractures 143
mastitis 135
meconium ileus 104
medical statistics 7, 130
medroxyprogesterone 106
Meissner's plexus 105
menorrhagia 42
Mental Health Act 1983 28
meralgia paraesthetica 58
meropenem 140
mesenteric adenitis 94
mesenteric ischaemia 61, 100, 104
mesenteric tears 66–7

metabolic acidosis
    compensated 100
    increased anion gap 100
metastatic bone pain 69
metatarsalgia 56
metformin-associated lactic acidosis 140
microbiology 5, 16, 52, 114
    encapsulated bacteria 140
migraine, abdominal 66
Monro-Kellie doctrine 134
Morton's neuroma/metatarsalgia 56
Muir and Barclay formula 25
multiple organ dysfunction syndrome 143
myeloproliferative disorder 96

nasoenteric fine-bore feeding 99
NCEPOD (National Confidential Enquiry into Perioperative
        Deaths) classification 61
necrotizing enterocolitis 104
negative predictive value (NPV) 149
Neisseria meningitidis 67
neonates 88, 127
    history, examination and assessment 127
    pyloric stenosis 106, 145–6
    see also paediatrics
neurogenic shock 136
neurological surgery 115
neurology 37
neuropathic pain 69
NICE guidelines, perioperative care 62
Nissen fundoplication 103
noradrenaline 98
null hypothesis 149
nutrition, see feeding
nutritional management 79, 84, 98

octreotide 67
oesophageal malignancy 93, 138
    Ivor Lewis procedure 26, 99, 104
    resection 26
oesophageal perforations 59
oesophageal stricture, benign 93
oesophagectomy, transhiatal 104
ophthalmological emergencies 30
osteomyelitis 68

p53 gene 96
paediatrics 88, 127
    consent issues 28
    fluid requirements 65
    history, examination and assessment 127
    see also neonates
palliative chemotherapy 26
pancreatic carcinoma 138
pancreatic disruption 64
pancreatic injuries 66

pancreaticoduodenectomy 132
pancreatitis, severe 140
papaverine 67
parenteral feeding 101–2
Parkland formula, fluid requirements 25
pathology 75
patient safety 117
PEG 26, 97
pelvic abscess 26
pelvic surgery 30
pelvirectal abscess 92
percutaneous endoscopic gastrostomy feeding (PEG) 26, 97
perianal abscess 92
perioperative care 73, 76, 79, 82, 112, 116, 119, 121, 123
    NICE guidelines 62
peritonitis, faecal 29
phaeochromocytoma 67
pharmacology 40
phenoxybenzamine 67
phenytoin, plasma levels, reduction of seizure level 29
photophobia 30
pilonidal sinus 106
planning investigations 83, 118
plantar fasciitis 21
pneumatosis intestinalis 104
pneumonectomies 94
pneumonia 24, 132
pneumothorax 39
polyglactin, suture 33
posterolateral thoracotomy 148
postoperative care 7, 73
    complications 4, 9, 14, 38
preoperative assessment and management 44, 46
prescribing 111, 120
prescribing, appropriate 13, 51, 54, 89
pressure-controlled intermittent mandatory ventilation 138
processus vaginalis 102
proctocolectomy 28
professional behaviour and leadership 43, 44
prostate cancer 105
prostatic hyperplasia 142
protein C and protein S deficiency 30
Proteus mirabilis 25
proto-oncogenes 96
pseudomembranous colitis 32, 132, 134
Pseudomonas aeruginosa 25
psychosomatic disease 66
pulmonary atelectasis 24
pulmonary embolism 24, 30
pulmonary oedema, secondary to fluid overload 61
pupillary constriction 30
purine and pyrimidine analogues, halting normal cell
    division 59
pyelonephritis 132–3, 143
    gentamicin 29
pyloric stenosis 106, 145–6

pyonephrosis 27
pyrexia, postoperative 24

quinolones 132

raccoon eyes 134
radial nerve lesions 23, 135–6
radiation enteritis 132
radioactive iodine-131 33
radiotherapy
    overall treatment time 33
    sealed sources 33
randomized controlled trial (RCT) 62
rectal tumours 98
recurrent laryngeal nerve damage 137
Redivac drain 108
Reiter's syndrome 21
renal failure 145
respiratory acidosis 100–1
respiratory problems 133–4
    ARDS 133–4
    CPAP 133
    IRV 133–4
    PCV 133
    PEEP 133
retroperitoneal haemorrhage 103
rheumatoid arthritis 63
    scleritis 30
risk management 139
Robinson drain 107
Roth's meralgia 58
Roux-en-Y reconstruction 69
Rutherford Morrison incision 69

sacroiliitis 21
saphenous vein graft 51
Saturday night palsy 23, 135
sciatic nerve lesions 58
scleritis 30
sclerosing cholangitis 63
sclerosing haemangioma 131
sebaceous cyst 131
shock, hypovolaemic 42
sickle cell disease 42, 61
sigmoid tumour 29
SIRS 5, 31, 52, 56, 136
skin lesions 109
skin, surgical conditions 2
skull fracture 134
small bowel follow-through 101
small bowel injury 58
small cell lung cancer (SCLC) 147
smoking cessation 143
somatization 66
Spearman rank correlation coefficient 26
spherocytosis 63

splenectomy 64, 67
splenic trauma 66
spondylolisthesis 20
sporicidal chemicals 34
squamous cell carcinoma 23
    anal canal 60
staghorn calculi 25
Staphylococcus aureus 31
sterilization (equipment) 19, 34
stoma, temporary vs permanent 28–9
'straight leg raise' test 20
Streptococcus pneumoniae 67
subdural haematoma 134–5, 144–5
surgical history and examination 3
surgical techniques 55
survival curves 26, 148
sutures
    absorbable 33
    silk 33
sutures (closures) 18, 33
syndesmophytes 20
systemic inflammatory response syndrome (SIRS) 5, 31, 52,
        56, 136

T-tube 108
tamoxifen 32, 33
tarsal tunnel syndrome 57
testicular teratoma 147
thalassaemia 63
thigh, lateral cutaneous nerve 57
thoracotomy
    absolute contraindications 95
    absolute indications 96
    clamshell 148
    fistula repair 95
    relative indications 95
    right posterolateral 147
thromboembolic disease, prophylaxis 30
thumb flexion, Froment's sign 23
thyroid surgery 137
Tinel's sign 57
TNM classification
    breast cancer 142
    lymph nodes 141
    malignant melanoma 141

malignant tumours 141
    renal cancer 141
tracheobronchial injury 59
tracheoesophageal fistula (TOF) 146
transfusion reactions 60
    anaphylaxis 60
    haemolytic 60
    iron overload 61
    pulmonary oedema secondary to fluid
        overload 61
trauma assessment and triage 39
    level of urgency 43
    resuscitation and early management 50
trauma (incl. multiple) 74, 86, 90, 113, 125
    assessment, triage 113
    children 90
    investigation 125
    management 125
    orthopaedics 1, 36
tumour cell DNA, anti-tumour antibiotics 60

ulcerative colitis 28, 56, 63, 68
ulnar nerve lesions 23, 136
urethral injury 145
urinary tract infections 27
    recurrence 53
urinary tract obstruction 143, 145
urosepsis, ESBL-related 140
uveitis, anterior 30

Valleix phenomenon 57
venous leg ulcer 96
venous thromboembolic disease 24
vertebral osteotomy 20
Virchow's node 93
visceral perforation 31
vomiting, cyclical vomiting syndrome 66

Wallace's Rule of Nines 24
Whipple's operation 132
Whiting's manoeuvre 106
wounds
    'clean contaminated' 31
    infections 31
    open 107